CHANGE *your body*

with the World's Fittest Couple

The Secret to a Great Body Revealed

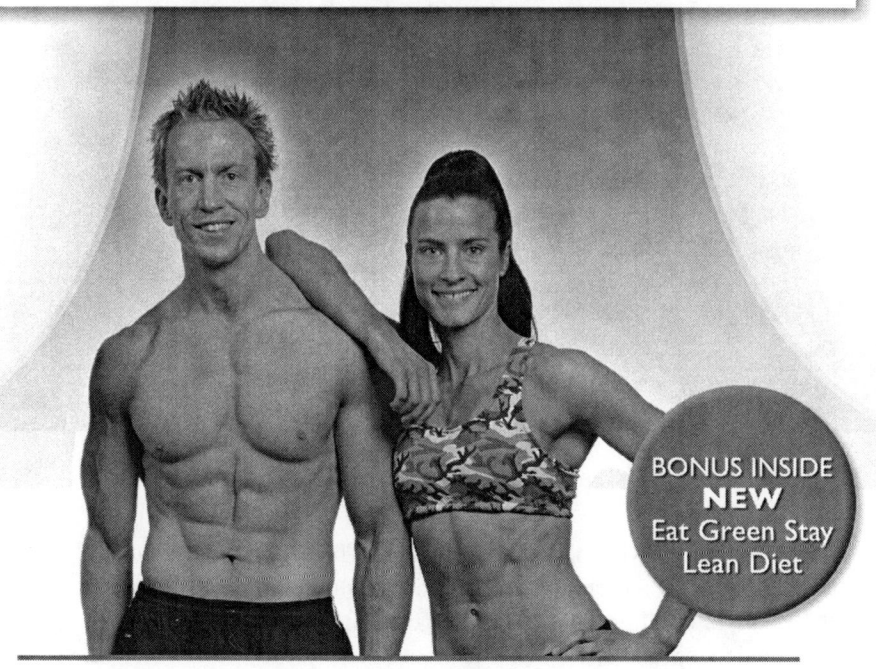

BONUS INSIDE
NEW
Eat Green Stay Lean Diet

Matt Thom & Monica Wright

All Rights Reserved
© MMVIII by Matt Thom & Monica Wright

This book may not be reproduced in whole or in part, by any means, without written consent of the publisher.

LIFESUCCESS PUBLISHING, LLC
8900 E. Pinnacle Peak Road, Suite D240
Scottsdale, AZ 85255

Telephone:	800.473.7134
Fax:	480.661.1014
E-mail:	admin@lifesuccesspublishing.com
ISBN:	978-1-59930-065-8
Cover :	Lloyd Arbour & LifeSuccess Publishing
Layout:	Lloyd Arbour & LifeSuccess Publishing

COMPANIES, ORGANIZATIONS, INSTITUTIONS, AND INDUSTRY PUBLICATIONS: Quantity discounts are available on bulk purchases of this book for reselling, educational purposes, subscription incentives, gifts, sponsorship, or fundraising. Special books or book excerpts can also be created to fit specific needs, such as private labeling with your logo on the cover and a message from a VIP printed inside. For more information, please contact our Special Sales Department at LifeSuccess Publishing.

"The best effect of any book is that it excites the reader to self activity".

—**Thomas Carlyle**, 1795 - 1881

"So much more than a fitness book, this information can be used to propel you forward in any area of your life; it is truly life changing. If you have a sincere desire to change your life, this book is a handbook that you'll use over and over again."

– **Bob Proctor**, *You Were Born Rich*,
and teacher on *The Secret*

Disclaimer

　　This book is written as a source of information only. It is solely for informational and educational purposes and is not medical advice. This book should by no means be considered a substitute for the advice of a qualified medical practitioner. Please consult a medical professional before commencing an exercise regime, nutritional plan, or changing your health habits. While the information contained in this book is the opinion of the authors, every effort has been made to ensure the accuracy of the information as of the date published. None of the statements in this book have been evaluated by the Food and Drug Administration (FDA) and are not intended to diagnose, treat, cure, or prevent any disease.

　　The authors and publishers disclaim all responsibility for any adverse effects, damages, or losses arising from the use of information contained in this book. Duplication of any part of this book is prohibited without prior permission from the authors.

Change Your Body with the World's Fittest Couple

Dedication

This book is dedicated to our amazing parents, family, and friends. These wonderful people all unconditionally supported two dreamers in their pursuit to increase the health and wellness of everyone around them.

This book is also dedicated to all our personal training clients who have inspired and challenged us over the last 15 years. Thank you for entrusting us with the most important thing in the world . . . your health.

Change Your Body with the World's Fittest Couple

Table of Contents

Foreword   11
Acknowledgments   17
Introduction   21
Section One – Get Motivated   27

    1. Don't Wait for a Second Chance   28
    2. Work Out Your Why   36
    3. It's All About YOU and Your Self-image   50
    4. You're Only as Good as Your Attitude   60
    5. Setting Goals   71
    6. Discipline   82
    7. Commitment   93
    8. Consistency and Creating Healthy Habits   100
    9. Overcoming Obstacles   104

Section Two – Become Educated   115

  10. Eat Yourself to Health   116
  11. Eat Green Stay Lean™   120
  12. The Importance of Water   155
  13. Supplements Make a Difference   165
  14. Eat Good Fats to Lose Fat   189
  15. Power Up with Protein   197
  16. What Carbohydrates to Eat   205
  17. Foods and Habits that Stop You from Losing Weight   213
  18. Mood Foods and Special Occasions   225
  19. Move It to Lose It   233

Section Three – Stay Dedicated   269

  20. Think Fit   270
  21. Our 15 Tips to Live By   293
  22. The 84 Day Body Challenge   301
  23. Eat Yourself to Health – Eating Plan   308
  24. Move It to Lose It – Exercise Plan   330
- Testimonials   336
- References   354

Matt Thom & Monica Wright

Foreword

I knew when I first met my husband, Matt, that my life would change forever. He had an energy and attitude about him that drew me in like an invisible force field. We met at Indian Head Summer Camp in Pennsylvania, U.S.A., on June 22, 1996. We were both summer camp counsellors to over 500 American children; I was running the gymnastic program, and he was teaching aussie rules, rugby and martial arts.

The summer camp lasted for nine weeks, and over this short time we developed a special bond. We fell in love and wanted to spend all our waking hours together. This attraction even got us in trouble with the camp's strict curfews and counsellor guidelines, but we didn't care. At the time, every minute was worth the risk. After the camp, we travelled around America for three amazing weeks. The experience of eating American food for 12 weeks was the turning point in our lives. We had never eaten so much processed food! I remember ordering a vegetarian pizza in a café and getting a pizza base with olives, onion, and cheese! The next time I ordered a vegetarian pizza, much to Matt's dismay, I asked the waitress if they could put chopped broccoli on the pizza, if I provided the broccoli. They said, "No problem." So, I headed out to the cooler in the car and came back with the broccoli.

My mum always served healthy meals at home, meals full of vegetables. So, it seemed completely alien to me to eat anything that wasn't served with salad or veggies. When I was living in Melbourne with my flatmate, Serena, she served baked bean toasted sandwiches for dinner one night. I immediately jumped up and quickly steamed a big bowl of broccoli for both of us. My sisters and Serena even presented me with a broccoli bouquet at my wedding.

I'm not sure what Matt thought of my obsession with broccoli and healthy eating, but it made us both realise how important eating a clean diet was for energy and maintaining a healthy weight. We both put on weight while in America, and on our return to Melbourne got straight back into our training and healthy eating. Matt started his personal training business, and I went straight into full-time gymnastic coaching at Loreto Mandeville Hall, Toorak.

I had been back in Australia for about 18 months when a friend suggested I try fitness competitions. I had never heard of them before, so I went along to watch a competition and was totally hooked! Getting up on stage was the challenge I had been looking for and it didn't seem that much different than gymnastics. My strength was the acrobatic fitness routine and I found that the weight training Matt was teaching me had really changed my body. I loved how I could manipulate food and training to achieve a muscular, toned body. When I walked out on stage in 1999 for the first time, I felt amazing and wanted to show everyone my acrobatic routine and inspire people to change their bodies. I won that first competition, with the biggest smile on my face. That was also the year Matt and I got married! I then went on to represent Australia in fitness competitions in America, England, and Europe from 1999 until 2006, winning a total of seven World Fitness titles.

Matt joined forces with me in 2002, to compete in the fitness pairs category in Germany at Fitness Universe. After competing on my own for so long, it was really fun to train, diet, and do a routine together.

I have wanted to be an author since I was 10 years old. So, in 2006, when Matt came up with the idea of writing a book together, I jumped at the chance. I remember documenting every gymnastic training session and competition I ever did when I was younger, and I remember nights of drawing up weekly charts in my bedroom to make sure I achieved my training and competition goals. The charts included things like making sure I got eight hours sleep, drinking water, practising my handstands, not eating junk food, doing my homework, and stretching.

I wouldn't call myself obsessed with checklists, but for every fitness competition in which I have competed, I've always had a checklist of things to do every day to achieve my goal. Matt and I have these checklists on our fridge, and we follow them for the 84 day lead-up to a competition. They are very effective in keeping us on track. Now we are bringing them to you through this book and our *84 Day Body Challenge Action Manual* which is sold separately.

Over the last seven years our involvement in fitness has been an amazing journey. We have learnt so much about the way the body works, have travelled all over the world, and have met some amazing athletes. Even though the training and diet is hard work, it taught us a lot about self-discipline, commitment, and time management. It has made us stronger, both physically and mentally.

Our last competition was June 2006 where we won our fourth World Fitness Pairs title, and I won my third Ms Fitness Universe title. This competition was our hardest ever because we filmed a documentary on our 84 day preparation to competition day. The pressure was on us to win again and we wanted to finish on top. The athletes we were up against were the toughest so far. The feeling of relief when we won our last competition was on par with our first win together in 2002, and we didn't sleep a wink all night from the adrenalin rush!

A major turning point for us was midway through 2005, when we were introduced to the powerful effects of following an alkaline diet. Up until then we had always followed a high protein diet and trained up to 2 hours every day to get ready for a competition, both of which produce acid in the body. We found in February 2006 that we were at our leanest ever and only two kilos off our stage weight, and we were in our off season!

We completely put this down to taking 30-60 ml of what we call *super juice* (a high antioxidant drink) plus 2 green whole food supplements – barley grass and spirulina on a daily basis. We also had alkaline foods such as spinach, broccoli, raw salads, vegetables, lemons, avocado, PiMag™ water, complex carbohydrates and nuts throughout the day, every day, with lean protein sources.

We didn't need to do the typical *body building diet* of training two hours a day anymore and going on a low carbohydrate, high protein diet to be lean. We breezed through the 84 day preparation for the competition and came in our leanest ever in 2006, eating a high alkaline diet. We had finally found the secret to a great body!

Now, I am at a point in my life where I have no competitions to prepare for. This is why I have decided to co-write this book with Matt.

We have written this book together, over the last two years, with many years of research, but for the ease of you, the reader; it has been written from Matt's perspective. It has been a huge project for both of us and all our spare time has been spent writing the book. So, as well as working together and living together, we now also spend all our spare time together. But, I wouldn't have it any other way. Matt's life experiences are inspirational, and we have both learned much about each other while writing this book. I hope you get inspired by Matt's story and knowledge just as much as I do on a daily basis.

Another reason we wrote this book was that we wanted to reach out and help more people. The obesity epidemic is out of control. By owning our own fitness training centre, we can really be there for people to educate and motivate them to change their bodies. However, there are too many people in the world who do not have this assistance. Our book is aimed at changing that. We are determined to put an end to this obesity epidemic by educating people and giving them the answers they need to live a happy and healthy life, full of wellness. Be part of the solution and join us on our health revolution.

What we have taught in this book, we have been doing with clients for the last 15 years. It is a proven system that has worked for them and will work for you. Refer to the testimonials at the back of the book, and find out what our inspirational clients have to say.

So . . . let's seize the day! Fit as much as you can into your 24 hours. Everyone has the same number of hours in a day; it is how you spend them that matters. My father always said to me, and I live by it every day, "Always go to sleep tired and not bored."

It is our goal to change your thinking through this book. Once you are hooked on thinking wellness, you will never look back!

Enjoy reading our book and please refer to our WEBSITE that is full of more helpful information at...

www.fitnesskick.com.au

Monica Wright

Ms. Fitness Universe (2002, 2003, and 2006)

Fitness Pairs Universe Champion (2002, 2003, 2005, and 2006)

Acknowledgements

To our parents... Ray, Jan, David, and Carol... YOU made us who we are today. Thank you, we love you.

To our brothers and sisters... Simm, Janette, Amanda, Rachelle, Sam, Dave, and Rob... thanks for being our pillars of strength and for all the amazing adventures we have had together!

To the children in our lives... Stella, Charli, Leni, Ruben, Hamish, Brylee, Kurtis ...thanks for the endless laughs and joy!

To Brent and Caz... for all your late night feasts and endless discussions on health and fitness and the amazing friendships we share.

To all the boys who are just like brothers for more than 20 years of friendship and adventure.

To Jonesy – A.K.A. Dr J – thanks for your faith, guidance, and constant support, you're a legend.

To our commercial agent and manager, Malcolm Twining... for helping us create a bigger picture and your faith in us from the very beginning!

Change Your Body with the World's Fittest Couple

To Jerome – A.K.A. Gloomus – thanks for being our first client!

To Kerry... thanks for being a straight shooter and telling us things we don't always want to hear, but need to know, and for your friendship.

To our dedicated coaches, who taught us discipline and skills in gymnastics and martial arts... Paul Hawkins (AFK), Liz, Margaret, Kath, and Mr. and Mrs. Langdon (PCYC Tasmania).

To the nurses at Royal Melbourne Hospital... thanks for your jokes, caring nature, and positive attitude that gave Matt strength to recover quickly.

To Fitness Kick @ Flemington trainers... thanks for helping us make a difference in people's lives. You guys are the best personal trainers in Australia!

To Brains and The Wizard... for introducing us to the wellness industry and your ongoing support and guidance.

To Travis and Belle... for inspiring us to think big!

To our accountants, Jason and Rob... you guys rock, the best accountants anyone could have.

To the amazing team at LifeSuccess Publishing USA and Morgan James Publishing... Bob Proctor, Liz Ragland, Autumn Drozda, Kandi Miller, Wendy Gallagher, Lloyd Arbour and Gerry Robert.

To Graeme Lancefield (NABBA/WFF) and Tony Lanciano (INBA) . . . thanks for all your great work in the fitness industry and your ongoing help and support.

To Troy Backhouse . . . thanks for your great designs and quick responses, wherever you happen to be in the world!

To Steven Pam . . . this book and *84 Day Body Challenge Action Manual* would not be the same without your photos!

To John Toomey . . . for being a great mentor and one of Australia's leading wellness experts. Your knowledge and passion is contagious!

To our sponsors for their belief, partnership, and commitment to helping us reach high levels of success.

And lastly to Ralph . . . our wonderful basenji dog!

Don't be Afraid of Life!
Don't Miss Smelling the Flowers
For Fear
You May Get Stung By A Bee!

—Author Unknown

Introduction

"A journey of a thousand miles begins with a single step."

—**Lao-Tze,** c. 604 BCE

Welcome to the journey that will change your life forever...

Today you are on your way to making positive changes to your health and fitness. Today you have made a decision to change and transform your body – and for that we congratulate you.

Just by picking up this book and reading it, you have made a conscious decision to improve your fitness, increase your energy levels, and above all, get motivated, become educated, and stay dedicated to look after your greatest asset... YOU.

We promise you that this book will give you the information and tools to change your body, which will ultimately change your life forever. The only way that you will not achieve results is if you stop reading. If you keep reading and apply our tips and knowledge, you will get results. Give up reading and you have given up on yourself. Keep reading and the book will never give up on you.

The sport of Fitness that we compete in, is a relatively new and developing sport, growing tremendously in the United States and Europe, particularly in the category of women's fitness. Pairs fitness started in the year 2000.

In Pairs Fitness competitions, there are two rounds: Round one is a 90-second fitness acrobatic routine, showcasing to the judges your cardiovascular, muscular endurance, agility, strength, power, flexibility, and showmanship. Round two is a muscularity round, or posing round, where up to 10 judges look at your body in eight compulsory poses. They judge the size and symmetry of the muscles on your body.

On the world stage, our bodies are required to look perfectly symmetrical with tightly toned muscularity and as little as 4% body fat for males and 15% for females. Now, to get into this shape, we follow a set training and eating regime for 84 days, and that is all it takes.

We have taught our training system, Fusion Workouts, and eating plan, Eat Green Stay Lean™, to thousands of clients over the last 15 years with an enormous amount of success. Our program gets results for our clients that commit to action. Meaning, that it's YOU who will be doing all the work. We will educate you and inspire you to take control of your health and turn that motivational switch on in your head!

Our training systems, outlined in this book, along with advice and recommendations, have been a continual work in progress over a 15-year period. This has been a combination of our passion in fitness and health and striving for excellence in our chosen sport. We have read literally hundreds of articles and books, listened to hundreds of motivational tapes and CDs, watched numerous documentaries, and surfed countless hours on the Internet viewing case studies and the latest research.

Change Your Body is a collection of research that has been done by inspiring authors, exercise specialists, wellness speakers, and others who are passionate about making a difference to the health of everyone on our planet. Without their knowledge, competing at the highest level and teaching others to change their bodies would not be possible. We acknowledge these people for helping not just us, but millions of people around the world.

We have gone through the trials and tribulations of all the latest exercise crazes and fads. We have tasted all the protein shakes, eaten the high-tech protein bars, and tried the revolutionary machines. Everything that has worked for us and our clients is here in this book in plain English for you to now devour!

Motivational comments, analogies, and stories will be spread throughout the book and will be found when you need them the most. The quotes in this book will also serve as daily motivators. Carry this book with you and flick through it on a daily basis for inspiring quotes, tips, and motivation.

Everything mentioned in *Change Your Body* is our opinion and what we believe to be true at the time we wrote it. The subject of health and fitness is an evolving one with new research being presented daily. We are the very best at what we do, and this book contains information that will put you in the best shape of your life.

Everyone's goals are different. Your goal may be to lose 5 or 20 kilograms, to increase muscle size, tone up or stop an addiction to junk food, sugar or even chocolate. Your goal may be to even compete in a sport at the highest level.

It doesn't matter. From now on, you don't need to worry about anything because we will give you all our knowledge and experiences to help you become the absolute best you can be. You have to take that first step and never look back, just keep on moving forward. No one else can do it for you. No time to exercise and eat healthy food? You will eventually have to find the time to be sick.

In over 15 years of personal training, we have seen thousands of clients, heard thousands of excuses, and experienced clients with countless body issues. We have the collective answers for you in this book. This book is a way we could reach and help many more people live a life with passion and be totally happy with how they look and feel. There are many books out there related to health and fitness and they promise to transform bodies. So, why is this one different?

The information you are about to read is responsible for everything we have achieved and it will change your body and your life, just like it did for us.

There is definitely a trend with today's diseases - cancer, diabetes, heart disease. They can all be prevented. Yes, prevented! Excess acidity in the body affects every one of us, because of the way we live, the way we eat, and the environment in which we live. The result is an internal acidic environment where disease can easily manifest, as opposed to a pH-alkaline environment which allows the body to function smoothly. Being alkaline is necessary for the body to resist disease. We will discuss more on this amazing acid-alkaline concept in our Eat Green Stay Lean™ chapter. This is one of the best ways to stay lean and healthy for the rest of your life, and something Monica and I follow 100%.

You must believe that you will have the body you always wanted. You are in control of what goes in your mouth. You are in control of your thoughts. Follow our Eat Green Stay Lean™ healthy eating plan and you will find your cravings will disappear, you will have more energy, and you will have a lean fit body. There are amazing supplements out there to help you make these changes easier, and we will educate you on these and how to use them.

Children's health has become a huge issue in Australia, with more than 50% of children being overweight and up to 30% being obese. Adult rates have also soared, with the number of overweight adults rising from 5.4 million to 7.4 million in 10 years. Education at a young age is the key to preventing this crippling health condition. But, it includes more than education. Adults are the key to saving their children. After all, adults are the role models for children and in general, children look up to and wish to resemble the adults in their lives. We should probably all ask ourselves who our children, our grandchildren, our nephews, our nieces, and our students are all looking up to as their role models. What mark are we leaving on their young and impressionable minds?

How unfortunate is it that we are leaving a legacy of poor health and obesity to our children. No one is born fat. They become fat. They learn from adults. Don't they deserve better? Now is the time to start teaching them healthy eating and daily exercise habits. Get healthy for the kids, do it for them!

As you can tell, this issue of childhood obesity is close to our hearts. We hope this book will kick-start many adults into leading healthier lives, and in doing so, create a better, healthier world for the children of today.

> *"Children have never been very good at listening to their elders, but they have never failed to imitate them."*
>
> —James Baldwin

Ultimately, remember to enjoy the journey to wellness and longevity, nothing is too hard, learn from your mistakes, and believe you can reach your destination.

Yours in Health and Fitness,

—Matt Thom and Monica Wright

SECTION I
GET MOTIVATED

Chapter 1

– Don't Wait for a Second Chance

"If you ever get a second chance in life, you've got to go all the way."

—Lance Armstrong

Imagine, for a moment, you had your life over again, what would you do differently?

As far as we know, we only get one life, one crack at it. So each and every one of us should be living and creating the life of our wildest dreams and aspirations.

The only way we can achieve our dreams and life purpose is by making the right choices in the food we eat, exercising every day, and reducing the toxins going into our bodies. To live a long, happy, healthy life is to be free of sickness and disease that only robs us of the life we want to live.

Chapter 1 — Don't Wait for a Second Chance

As a good friend of mine, Brent Lavery, likes to say, "Once you are dead, you are dead, so you may as well go for it." It's not hard; it is all about knowledge and choice. YOU choose the life you want to live and how you want to feel every day.

There are not a lot of people on this planet who can say they have miraculously escaped death and have been given a second chance at life. I am a member of the second chance club. I should be dead, but through what can only be described as a miracle, I am alive to tell my tale.

My story is exactly that, a story. I am not here to preach to you and tell you what you should and shouldn't be doing. It's just what Monica and I have done. By sharing our experiences, it may help others to live a happy, healthy and long life.

Waking up in intensive care at the Royal Melbourne Hospital on Monday morning February 12, 2001, was one of the most surreal experiences of my life. Earlier that week, I was living my normal life running a thriving mobile personal training business working with approximately 50 clients per week. Everything they did I did: every push-up, every hill sprint, and every kilometre I was right there beside them. My clients ranged from unconditioned housewives to athletes. I am amazed at how much training I did during those early days, but it was worth every minute. It worked and I got results because I was willing to do every exercise I asked them to do. Some weeks I ran a total of 120 kilometres, rode 200 kilometres, and swam four kilometres, plus weights and conditioning. I had a reputation of being tough and getting results with any client.

At the time, I trained my wife, Monica, to compete in and win two state fitness titles which qualified her to compete in Ms. Fitness

World in Las Vegas in 2000. She finished in 13th place. This was the best-placed Australian effort at the time. These results made my personal training business boom, I had a waiting list and started making plans to open my own fitness centre.

As well as training with my clients, I was also training for an hour and a half every day to compete in my first state open martial arts tournament, scheduled to be held in April 2001. The massive changes I made in my life were starting to unfold exactly the way I had planned. Incredible as it seemed, only a few years earlier I was working a desk job, went out most nights, was overweight, and was the most unfit I had ever been. I literally could not run 200 metres without stopping and being completely out of breath.

The past was gone and I never looked back, my life was awesome. I was in love with my beautiful, fit wife, loved my business which I had built up since 1996, and was the fittest I had ever been. Yes, life couldn't really get that much better; unfortunately it was about to get much worse. The following story of my train accident is told by my wife Monica, as I was unconscious and have no recollection of the accident. My first memory is waking up in the hospital.

The Train Story

Matt and I were both on our way home from a Sunday afternoon bike ride on February 11, 2001. He always rode faster than me, but would continually do u-turns and ride back to me or wait for me at the lights to catch up. It was 8:30 at night, just going on dusk and I was about 50 metres behind Matt.

I saw him cross the railway crossing ahead of me, and then, all of a sudden, it seemed like his bike collapsed under him and he was on

Chapter 1 — Don't Wait for a Second Chance

the tracks. I started pedalling faster to find out what happened, and when I got closer to the crossing, I could see he was not moving and was entangled underneath his bike. It was then that I heard the crossing lights start to go and the boom gates lower. I pedalled faster, threw my bike down, and ran under the boom gates to get to the other side of the tracks where Matt lay. I vividly remember seeing Matt's upper body lying right on the tracks, seeing the lights of the train coming up about 100 metres away, and knowing I had seconds to pull him off the tracks.

I reached forward to grab his shirt with both my hands and pulled, but because he had a thin cheesecloth shirt, it tore at the shoulder and I fell back. I got up to try a second time but had to leap out of the way of the train as it thundered through the crossing, hitting Matt.

The next few seconds in my mind are like slow motion, and even now, I am very emotional and anxious as I write. I remember yelling out and watching as the train hit and propelled him and his bike up into the air, higher than the train itself, and Matt landing about 40 metres away, smashing against a concrete pylon. I didn't think, at anytime, that he was dead, or had been sliced in half by the train. I could see a whole body lying on the ground, as well as a lot of blood and dirt, and Matt still tangled up in his bike.

I ran as fast as I could to his side and grabbed his hand yelling, "Matt squeeze my hand if you can hear me!" over and over again. A lady, who witnessed the accident, came up and put her hand on my shoulder and said, "Let him go, there's not much you can do, he's been hit by a train, he's dead."

She tried to pull me off him, but I kept yelling, "Squeeze my hand if you can hear me," and told her to ring the ambulance, and asked if she had any blankets or towels to help stop the blood. The train stopped about 50 metres away after the collision, and I remember people hanging out of the windows looking at me.

I prayed continuously for him to be okay, and then finally, Matt squeezed my hand and opened one of his eyes. His face was covered with blood and he asked, "What happened?" I told him he had fallen off his bike and got hit by a train. Because of his massive leg injuries, he had no feeling in his legs, and he asked me if his legs were all there. That was the first time I looked down to the tangled wreck of his legs and bike and could see that the bike had been embedded into his leg. I grabbed the towels to stem the blood.

I asked him not to speak anymore because I could see a lot of his teeth had fallen out and I didn't want him to swallow any. I sat with him, holding his head and hands. The ambulance arrived within minutes.

They wanted to know his name, age, address, who I was, and whether he was allergic to anything. They took over and looked after his injuries. The transit police arrived and I had to give a statement. We went over to the tracks with a flashlight where Matt had fallen, and saw there was blood on the ground, and about five massive potholes around the train tracks. The blood had come from the side of his face and temple where he had hit the ground knocking himself out after hitting one of the potholes. I made a mental note to come back the next day to take photos of the potholes and blood, as evidence.

They had Matt on a stretcher, and I held his hand as they put him in the ambulance. I noticed that his wedding ring, which he wore

Chapter 1 — Don't Wait for a Second Chance

on a necklace, was gone. I quickly searched the area with a flashlight, but could not find the ring or necklace. I sat in the front and travelled with him to the hospital. I regard myself as an emotional person because any movie can make me cry, but I had still not shed a tear. It must have been shock. On the way to hospital, I rang Matt's brother, Simm, and his mum, Jan, and remember saying, "Matt is okay, but he just got hit by a train." They came to the hospital straight away.

I couldn't go into the emergency room while they were treating Matt because it all got a bit too much, so I sat in a small waiting room while Simm and Jan went in to be with him. That is when what actually happened really hit me. The vivid images kept coming back into my mind and the tears flowed; I visited the toilet many times to be physically sick.

With Matt's injuries cleaned and bandaged, I went in to be with him as they rolled him into the intensive care unit. He had over 80 stitches on his face, lost four teeth, broke toes, had a deep laceration 30 centimetres long on his left leg down to the bone, and major damage to both his knees. He also had a neck brace on until all x-rays had been done on his neck and spine.

"Where there is great love there are always miracles."

—Willa Cather

On that Monday morning, 18 hours after the accident, opening my eyes to see my wife, family, and closest friends staring at me is a memory I will never forget.

Their faces were white as clouds with shocked expressions, and at that point, I didn't know what exactly was happening. Monica then conveyed to me the details of what had happened. I lay there a little dazed and confused, trying to process what I had just been told. Looking out to all the closest people in my life, I felt like my world had just been flipped upside down.

Here I was, lying in hospital with a banged-up body, a face almost unrecognisable, and in a state of shock. In this fragile state, you would think my friends would be nurturing and supportive . . . no, not my mates. I remember hearing things like:

Jonesy, "Come on, get up mate, stop acting, you are not that bad."

Pearcey, "Mate, I would kiss you, but you are just too ugly."

Within about two minutes, they had lifted the mood in the room from silence to joy and laughter.

It's always the people that you are closest to in life that manage to keep you grounded, challenge you when you need it, and love and support you unconditionally. I am extremely fortunate to have a loving family and my close group of mates who are more like brothers than friends.

Chapter 1 — Don't Wait for a Second Chance

From that morning, with the laughing and comments flying around, I was determined to make a speedy recovery so I could be with my family and friends once again.

Eighteen months after my accident, Monica and I represented Australia at the 2002 WFF Fitness Universe Championships in Germany in the Fitness Pairs Division. We won and became the only husband and wife team to win the World Fitness Pairs title. In the years to follow, Monica and I went on to win another three World Fitness Pairs titles and we became the most successful Australian couple to compete in the sport of fitness.

This is the basis of my story of how I began the journey through rehabilitation to the world stage, how I felt about the incident which changed my life, the overpowering feelings of love and emotion that empowered me to take charge and to motivate myself to become the best I could be!

I hope my story will motivate you because the aim of this book is to help empower you to change your body, which will change your life. It took being hit by a train to change my life. You can do it by reading this book, which will be just as effective and much less painful.

Chapter 2

– Work Out Your Why

*"To get the body in tone,
get the mind in tune."*

—Zachary T. Bercovitz, 1895 - 1984

The first section of this book is titled Get Motivated. In Chapter I – A Second Chance, we wanted to share with you an event that changed both our lives for the better . . . yes, that's right, for the better!

Wherever you are in life regarding your health, know this: It does not matter. It is only a starting point. Everyone has the potential to change their lives for the better; there is no one alive who is beyond help. The following chapters in this section are all essential ingredients for you to get motivated to change your body.

Chapter 2 — Work Out Your Why

But, before we get into a serious sweat and start steaming a kilo of broccoli, this chapter is to work out your WHY. Why do you want to change your body?

Through our experience, everyone's "why" is different. Work out YOUR why before you go any further. Without a why, you will start and most likely drop off.

You must understand that working out your "why" is your driving force, your source of inspiration that you can draw upon when times get a little tough – and we promise you that everyone's journey is a roller coaster ride of emotional highs and lows. The world we live in has a massive amount of outside pressures, distractions, obstacles, and challenges, so you need to keep your mind focused on your WHY.

Every single client we have ever trained has come to us because they have wanted to change their bodies. In almost every case, they have told us, in the same sentence, that they already know what they should be doing to change their bodies. They want to change, and they know what they need to be doing. So, why are they not doing it?

When asked why they want to change, or why they aren't doing what they should be doing, it is usually because they do not have a definite, or strong enough reason.

Usually, it takes most of us hitting rock bottom, or developing an illness, or getting to a point where we say, "Right, that's enough, never again, I am finished with that." When we add enough emotion, we can make a change, just like that. But, why do we have to reach that point?

It's because most of us are like the dog in the following story which beautifully illustrates my point:

A man walks past a house where a dog is lying on the porch moaning in great pain.

The man asks the dog's owner, "Why is he moaning so badly? What is wrong with him?" The owner tells the man that the dog is lying on a nail. The man questions why the dog isn't moving.

The owner looks down at the dog and says, "It's not hurting him bad enough to move, it's just hurting him enough to moan and groan about it."

Most people do the same. They would rather moan and whine about what's wrong with them, without doing anything about it. They only truly decide to change their lives when enough is enough – when they can't take it anymore.

—Author Unknown

Over the years of training clients, the most common whys we have heard are:

- Sickness or ill health – through a combination of poor lifestyle choices they have found themselves told by the medical profession that if they don't change what they are doing, then they will end up in hospital, or in the ground!
- Outside pressure – from family, or a loved one who wants them to change to be around a lot longer, because they understand

Chapter 2 — Work Out Your Why

the importance of physical and mental health which works to increase longevity.

- Getting married – a classic motivator, a photo that you are going to have for the rest of your life, this is a powerful motivator and a great short-term why.

- Having children – if you could harness the energy that children have, you would have enough power to run a small country. So, when the why becomes "I need to do it for my kids to set a good example for them and to have the energy to play with them," this is a very powerful why and the strongest motivator.

- Can't fit into clothes anymore – this is a huge drop in self-image when you get ready to go out and can't fit into your clothes anymore! If you don't start exercising or eating better you will have to buy a new wardrobe! Your better and cheaper option would be to start moving your body, start saying no, and eating wholesome foods to fit into your favourite clothes again. Do not take the option of hiding your body in bigger clothes.

- Me – I need to do this for me. It's my body. It's where I live and I am sick and tired of being sick and tired. This is the best why out of all of the above because healthy eating and exercise is one of the only things you can do for YOU. Think about it, a lot of the time you are doing things for others, and you put yourself last. STOP! It's time you were number one. Do it for you. If you truly believe you are worth it, you can and will achieve anything you want.

So, it's time for YOU to think about WHY you need to change. Once you have decided, write it down or start a separate journal for your thoughts. Be as honest as you can. It's time to get serious and find your motivation to become a healthier YOU.

To help with this we have outlined our whys below. It is really about understanding your own personality and what motivates you to take action.

Monica's Why

People always ask me, "How do you find the motivation to exercise and eat healthy every day?" For me, it is not a chore. It is a habit that I have been doing all my life. My mum was a Physical Education teacher and Dad would bike ride every day, so we grew up in a healthy, active household. My twin sister, Amanda, my older sister, Janette, and I had to walk to and from school every day – we lived on top of a huge hill in Tasmania, so it was not easy! Physical Education was my favourite subject in school, and I participated in all sports throughout my school life, and competed in gymnastics. I grew up knowing that being active kept me healthy and gave me energy. It made me feel good, it was fun, and I just assumed that everyone was this active!

I competed in gymnastics from ages 4 to 19. I never had a weight problem because I was so active and Mum always served us healthy food. Water was the only beverage of choice. I remember being allowed to buy lunch at school only once a month because most of it was junk and Mum would prefer us to eat healthy food. So, when I left home at 18, my body was used to eating wholesome, healthy food, and I never craved chocolate or junk food. My parents had pretty much set me up with awesome healthy eating habits. Thanks guys!

One thing I realised, was the direct connection between exercise and food. When I stopped gymnastics at age 19, I still continued eating the same foods and ultimately gained weight. So, I joined my first gym, started doing classes, weights, yoga, kickboxing, running, and I

Chapter 2 — Work Out Your Why

maintained a good weight all year. It is now embedded in my brain that there is no way that you can eat and not exercise!

I still love high-calorie foods every now and then, such as alcohol or a piece of cake, but I always make sure I don't overdo it and that it is worth having. I pack my day with getting lots done at work or home and training hard, and then I can sit back and really enjoy that glass of wine! Having the mindset of training every day makes me think about what sort of training I will do tomorrow, and that relates to what I do the night before. It is easy to moderately drink and eat good food when you look forward to training the body the next day. If you have ever tried training after having a big night out drinking, or eating too much the night before, then you know it is not enjoyable at all!

For me, training every day, whether it is a power walk, yoga, a bike ride, a run, kickboxing, gymnastics, hiking, swimming, weights, it is time for ME. I find solutions to any problems I have when I train, and it makes me feel invigorated and alive!

If you don't move your body, then of course you are going to put on weight and be flabby. I love going out for meals, preparing a big feast, and the taste of amazing food . . . just ask Matt. I haven't met anyone who does not like tasty food! Why then do people choose not to exercise? If you are putting too much into your body, but not MOVING your body then you will have a weight problem! One of our clients only trains so he can enjoy Italian food every day! That is his why.

If I sat on my butt every day, I know I would be tired and put on weight. Exercise and healthy food give me energy. I do not want to be overweight. I love having a fit body and wearing any clothes I like. I use exercise to have time out for ME. When I am busy with work, I always combine two things together so I am doing incidental exercise such as:

- Walking to work instead of driving
- Running or walking with my dog, Ralph
- Walking to the shops and carry my shopping home
- Doing push-ups and sit-ups during commercial breaks
- On any car trip, getting dropped off early from my destination and running or walking the rest of the way

Guaranteed, if you go away with me, I will always be organizing some physical activity to do. I am not one to sit around and do nothing. I remember one time while sailing with a group of friends in Queensland, we all decided to jump in the dinghy and go over to an island for a hike. I said I would swim from the boat across to the island instead – about 600 metres – and coaxed a couple of others to come with me. Anyway, to cut a long story short, we found out later that the particular inlet we had swum across was a breeding ground for hammerhead sharks!

So my WHY is that I actually love training and eating healthy; it keeps me lean which makes me feel great, and I am setting up a healthy body so I can fight off any disease that comes my way.

Matt's Why

I briefly mentioned in the introduction that I haven't always been fit, healthy, or in shape. It was about 10 years before the train accident that I was on a path of self-destruction.

At the time, I was at university studying exercise science. For the ultimate contradiction, I wasn't exactly practicing what I was learning – in fact, I was doing just the opposite. While I was completing a Bachelor of Applied Science, I was also completing a Bachelor of Drinking at most of the local watering holes.

To give you a little insight into the most social years of my life, I was voted by my fellow peers to be Physical Education Society Social President in my first year of university. I kept this role for three years. As I look back at the university days, it was mostly a juggle between cramming and partying. I had my excuses - my parents at the time had separated, I was living out of home, and I used getting drunk as an escape. During my days at the university, I put myself into a poor health state where I was overweight and the most unfit I have ever been. This reminds me of an old Chinese proverb which certainly rings true for me:

> *"Before the age of 30, Man chase disease, but after the age of 30, disease chases Man"*

So why am I telling you this? It is because the biggest excuse or cop-out I have heard to this day when I am pushing clients really hard is, "It's alright for you, you're fit, it's easy for you. You don't understand how hard it is!"

It was like I was one of the lucky ones born fit and they were one of the unlucky ones born fat, and we came from two different worlds, and how could I relate to what they are going through? Let's dispel a few myths. Nobody is born fit or fat. If someone is fit, it's because they have worked hard at it through being disciplined in training and diet, by putting themselves first, exercising, and saying no to that chocolate cake. By the same token, if someone is overweight, it didn't happen because of one poor decision. It has happened progressively over a period of time due to poor health choices they made on a consistent basis.

Now, I have always been a fairly competitive person . . . okay a very competitive person. So, my why in regards to health and fitness has always been competition-based, and for me, it is a great motivator. Challenge me, bet me, or even dare me, and I will do everything in my power to win. Now, for me, this comes from having a very competitive father who used to race dune buggies and was a three-time Australian champion. So, growing up in his house with a younger brother and an older sister, everything was a competition. This win-at-all-costs mentality is heavily ingrained in my personality, and it's a driving force.

Just prior to my train accident, I was undoubtedly the fittest I had ever been. I was heavily involved in martial arts in my late teens and kept it up well into my twenties.

In 1996, after meeting Monica in a summer camp in America where I was teaching martial arts to hundreds of American kids, I met Paul Hawkins, who became my new martial arts instructor and mentor. He is the Shihan Master of Australian Freestyle Kickboxing – a style he put together from 12 different fighting forms, designed purely for the street. At the time, he was a Tasmanian police officer and Head Tactical Trainer of the Special Operations Group.

After studying under him for five years, and working my way up the ranks, he entered me into the Open Martial Arts Tournament. I had a goal and trained hard. It was a tournament I wanted to win. The tournament was to be held in April 2001, and I had been training very hard for 12 months.

Chapter 2 — Work Out Your Why

After a training bike ride on February 11, 2001, I woke up in the hospital. That week in the hospital was, to date, the hardest of my life, both emotionally and physically. I still felt like the same person on the inside. I still felt motivated, energetic, and a little hyperactive, just as I had the day before. But I was trapped in a body that wasn't the same. It was all busted up and didn't work properly.

The two were now out of sync. My body did not do what my mind wanted. The inability to move freely was a realization that I was not ready for mentally.

There I was, lying completely still in the hospital bed with a neck brace, leg brace, and bandages all over, staring at the white ceiling and trying to comprehend what had happened and find out what my exact injuries were. It was very difficult at the time and was made even worse by observing the faces of concerned medical staff as they wheeled the bed from intensive care down to a dark basement where big machines did test after test on my banged-up body. In the hospital, it's the other senses that really start to take over and start painting a mental picture or image in the brain – watching peoples' expressions, hearing whispers from doctors and nurses, the look in the eyes of family and friends and the sounds and smells of everyday living in the intensive-care high-dependency ward.

I remember one night lying there in the dark listening to the patient in the next bed die. The machines started beeping as the person let out gasps and splutters – a loud combination of air rushing out of the lungs and a snort, described as the death rattle. It is the most horrid sound I have ever heard. I pressed my panic button and moments later nurses came running in and attended the person, but there wasn't anything they could do. At that moment, death became very real. Was I going to be the next to die? I felt, for the first time, that my life was out of my hands.

45

A week later, I was out of hospital, recouping at home and reality had truly set in! I had been told by doctors and physios that I would never run again and the activities I could do would be limited for the rest of my life. I hit rock bottom, was very moody, losing hope and becoming depressed.

At the time, I was unbearable to live with. I had lost all motivation, was negative, and, once again, I turned to alcohol as an escape. I was still unable to work and my clients were waiting patiently for me to return, and I did not know if this was possible. My relationship with Monica became strained because I did nothing but feel sorry for myself. I felt I did not have much to look forward to.

At home, I was still getting a few visitors, and I would put on a brave, cheery face; but on the inside, I just wanted to be left alone. Good friends of mine, Jemima and Dave, dropped off a couple of books for me to read: *Awaken the Giant Within* by Anthony Robbins and *You Were Born Rich* by Bob Proctor. I had never read any personal development books or motivational books before, so over the next few weeks, I began reading these books and started to focus and become more positive. I started to think differently and started to think of what I could do. I needed to set a goal and it didn't need to be health or exercise-related. I had accepted my situation and wanted to focus on something new. I became motivated again.

After discussing what I could do with Monica, she came back about a day later and pitched a goal to me that was cunning and smart – and I played right into her hands. You see, Monica knew what made me tick and knew my personality traits better than anyone, and she challenged me in a way that no one else has ever done.

If I remember correctly, it went a little like this:

"Honey, I have a great idea that would be a lot of fun, but you probably won't be able to do it. It might be too hard for you."

"What's that babe?" I replied.

"Well, you know how I really want to compete at the WFF Fitness Universe in Germany next year?"

"Yes," I said

"Well, you know how you will be training me and coming over anyway, I just thought . . . oh don't worry about it, it's impossible, you just couldn't do it!"

"Couldn't do what?" I replied, now really wanting to know what this impossible challenge was.

"Well they have a fitness pairs division at the Fitness Universe, and I thought we could train and do it together; but maybe the year after. It's just not enough time to get ready for a World Competition."

Now, a little intrigued and nibbling at the worm on the hook, so to speak, I asked, "Well, how long before the competition?"

"It's only 18 months, do you think you could do it?" she asked.

"YES!" Bang! She got me, hook, line, and sinker. She pitched to my competitive side, my ego, challenging me right after reading two very powerful books, with the bottom line "You can do anything you put your mind to."

The timing was perfect and delivered beautifully. Now I had a WHY! How I was going to do it did not matter because now I had a WHY, and it was all my idea, wasn't it? My wife is brilliant!

Not liking your body and wanting to be leaner is not enough. Get a Why that is so strong that it serves you like a ship's rudder, keeping you on course even when the seas become rough.

If you can't think of a single WHY then stop reading, and keep doing what you are doing. If you don't have that source of motivation to draw upon when times get tough, then you will quit. Understand that we put ourselves last. We live in incredible times on planet Earth, and never have we been more time-poor, more stressed out, or lived lives with more pressure, uncertainty, and worry. Working out a why in today's world should be easy. Just think of how many people you know who are overweight, even obese, and have diabetes or cancer. We all know people who can improve their health, but before we can help them, we need to start with ourselves.

The only way we can change the current statistics and alarming disease rate is one person at a time. So, it is your choice: choose disease or choose life. Exercise and eating healthy are a couple of things in life you can do for your own health and vitality.

Chapter 2 — Work Out Your Why

What Life is About

"There was once an emperor who told his horseman that he could have as much land as he could ride across on one horse. The horseman quickly jumped onto his horse and rode as fast as possible to cover as much land area as he could. He kept on riding and riding, whipping the horse to go as fast as possible. Even when he was hungry or tired, he did not stop because he wanted to cover as much area as possible.

It came to a point when he had covered a substantial area and he was exhausted, and was dying. Then he asked himself, "Why did I push myself so hard to cover so much land area? Now I am dying and I only need a very small area to bury myself."

—**Author Unknown**

Chapter 3

– It's All About YOU and Your Self-image

You can be whatever type of person you choose to be. Your habits, your behaviours, your responses . . . all your choice!

Having ascertained your why, or purpose for changing your body, you now have a starting point and source of motivation. Remember *you* are an investment! So anytime you spend money on healthy food, supplements, gym memberships, or personal trainers, you are investing in YOU.

Chapter 3 — It's All About YOU and Your Self-image

Nobody can exercise for you, or eat healthy for you; it's you that has to do it. You are the only one that has to live your life. So, forget about the past – what's done is done. Yesterday is gone forever, but you must accept responsibility for where you are now. The day you take complete responsibility for yourself is the day you stop making excuses. That's the day you start on the road to success.

Now, let's prepare for the future. Cherish your good memories and learn from the challenges. You have the power to succeed at anything and do things you never thought you could do. But before you start on a path of action, what do you think about YOU?

During my rehabilitation after the train accident, I was at a point in my life where I had to turn inward and put myself first. It was hard at the beginning because for the previous five years my business revolved around helping others achieve their goals. My goal was to help them achieve their success. Now that I had a goal for the World Fitness Pairs Title, the focus was on getting my body back to a point of proper function. So, initially it was all about rehabilitation.

I spent at least four hours a day working on rehabilitation, working with doctors and physiotherapists. After years of giving, I found spending this much time on me very difficult. I actually hated every minute of rehabilitation because it was slow, tedious, and painstaking to learn to do things again that only a week earlier I could do without giving a second thought. Now, it took all my energy and concentration just to do simple things like bending my knees to sit in a chair. The only thing that kept me focused was my goal of winning a World Fitness title. I was the only one who could do it, no one else could do my rehabilitation for me, and once I realised this, I saw that the more I focused on me, the more progress I made. For the first time in years, I was my number one priority – and it felt good!

I have a client who is a very successful businessman. He is very astute at financial matters. When I first met him, money seemed to be the most important aspect of his life. I noticed he wasn't working up to his potential. In his training sessions, he was not focused; he went through the motions without really giving it 100%. It was clear to me that his health was not as important to him as money.

So, to get my point across, I asked him if he had a retirement plan. He looked at me like I was stupid and assured me of his financial security. I then told him that it was a shame he would not be around to enjoy it. I was able to convey to him that health should be the most important component of his retirement plan, for without his health, no amount of money mattered.

As soon as he understood that his health was his greatest investment, he stepped up to the challenge and worked hard to be the fittest and healthiest that he had ever been. The fitter and healthier he got, the more his business flourished. He realised that exercise and eating well were perfect companions to his work life. They went hand in hand; the exercise was a great stress relief, while healthy eating gave him the extra energy he needed to run a successful business. Your health is your best retirement plan. Without it, you won't be able to live any kind of fulfilling life.

So, what motivates you? Are you motivated by spending time with your family, living to your fullest potential or feeling your best? Why have you, all of a sudden, decided to change your life? With the increased risk of diabetes, heart disease, cancer, and the obesity epidemic plaguing the world, your best defence is to change not just your body, but your mind as well.

Chapter 3 — It's All About YOU and Your Self-image

Everyone has an image, in their mind, of what they would like to look like and what they would like to do. This image of how you see yourself is an important starting point. It is necessary to have a positive self-image, if you are to undertake this fitness journey.

> *"We are what we think. All that we are arises with our thoughts. With our thoughts, we make our world."*
>
> **—Buddha**

Everything that has ever been made, and every human achievement that has been accomplished, started as a single thought. So, remember that every thought you have, could in fact, become reality. Start thinking of what you really want your life to be like.

When you can see yourself in better shape, or finishing a fun run, or winning a competition, you will start to feel the happiness and accomplishment. It is important to remember that when you add emotion to a goal it becomes more real.

Do you get excited when you think of a holiday coming up, or a day off? That is because you imagine what you are going to do, and holidays are always joyful and stress free, and so are days off. You need to get into the same mindset when you imagine having the body you want, and being healthy and stress free. Keep picturing these amazing images in your head and you will start to live them. Your mind does not know the difference between what is real and what is not real. So, why not fill your mind with what you want to be?

Your Self-Image

Self-image is how you see yourself in relation to others. This may be how you see yourself physically or it may be more about the idea you have of yourself. It is very important because it affects your self-esteem and confidence. Your self-image includes:

- **What you think you look like physically**
- **How your personality comes across**
- **What kind of person you think you are**
- **What you think others think of you**

If you have a poor image of yourself then your self-esteem will be poor. How exactly are they different? Self-esteem focuses on how you feel about yourself. Self-image is about how you see yourself. They are, as you can see, very close.

Your self-image plays a big role in your ability to change. Where you are in your life is an outcome of your thinking. You can never outperform your self-image. A positive self-image is imperative and starts on the inside. You must break down old negative beliefs and destructive habits. Once you become focused, healthy habits will form and you will gain self-confidence and a good self-image. I remember staring at myself in the mirror after I was released from the hospital. I saw a stranger looking back at me who had two missing front teeth and a face full of bruises and cuts. I was deeply conflicted. On the inside, I was still this fit and healthy guy, while on the outside, I felt like a monster. My negative self-image kept me from wanting to recover and recapture my life.

Chapter 3 — It's All About YOU and Your Self-image

If you look in the mirror and you don't like what you see, nobody else is responsible for that. You are. So, if you don't like it, change it. To a large extent your life is what you make it. Nothing will happen by itself.

If you think you look a certain way, then your mind will start to accept your thought as a reality. Once I decided that my self-image was positive, I was able to overcome enormous obstacles. Don't tell yourself that you are fat and need to go on a diet because your mind is accepting your image as reality. More than likely, you will not lose weight because you believe that you are fat. It is important to remember that nothing happens overnight. Don't focus on quick fixes or fads. Focus on healthy eating, exercise, and a positive self-image. You will begin to see remarkable changes occur.

"A Native American tells about a brave who found an eagle's egg and put it into the nest of a prairie chicken. The eaglet hatched with the brood of chicks and grew up with them.

All its life, the eagle, thinking it was a prairie chicken, did what the prairie chickens did. It scratched in the dirt for seeds and insects to eat. It clucked and cackled. And it flew in a brief thrashing of wings and flurry of feathers no more than a few feet off the ground. After all, that's how prairie chickens were supposed to fly.

Years passed, and the eagle grew very old. One day, it saw a magnificent bird far above in the cloudless sky. Hanging with graceful majesty on the powerful wind currents, it soared with scarcely a beat of its strong golden wings.

*'What a beautiful bird!' said the eagle to its neighbour, 'What is it?'
'That's an eagle – the chief of the birds,' the neighbour clucked.
'But don't give it a second thought. You could never be like him'.
So, the eagle never gave it a second thought, and it died thinking
it was a prairie chicken."*

—Author Unknown

Your self-image is also decided by how people perceive you, and this will affect how they relate to you. It can affect your relationships either positively or negatively. Don't listen to society's view about what a self-image should be. Make your mind focus on what you want to be, not what society wants you to be. Your view of yourself is shaped by your unique thoughts and beliefs. If you let others dictate your beliefs then you will have a distorted view. No one but YOU is responsible for deciding who you are!

How to Improve your Self-image

- Write down things you like about yourself – include your appearance, personality, and skills.
- Realise that you are going to have negative thoughts and don't beat yourself up about them. Take a deep breath and imagine yourself in new clothes, running in a fun run. It is impossible to think positive all the time. Every person on the planet has negative thoughts. Realise this and just don't focus on them.
- Eat healthy and exercise – you will feel better and look better! Only listen to the good things people have said about you, and write them down, if you desire.

Chapter 3 — It's All About YOU and Your Self-image

- Ask yourself whether or not your view of yourself is accurate and examine why you see yourself like you do.
- Make any changes you think would help you. For example: clothes, appearance, hairstyle, and behaviour in certain situations.
- Accept things about yourself that are true and learn to think about them in a positive way.
- View criticism in a constructive way and learn from it.
- Don't be limited by your self-image; step outside of it and break free – it doesn't have to control you or keep you down. Changing your behaviours will change how others see you and will also help to change your own attitude toward yourself and your abilities.
- Accept new challenges positively.
- Read self-help books. Three of my favourites include Awaken the Giant Within by Tony Robbins, You Were Born Rich by Bob Proctor, and Maximum Achievement by Brian Tracey. You are only limited by your efforts and confidence! Believe in yourself!

I had a client, Vicki, who was an extremely vibrant and tenacious woman. Vicki had a very destructive self-image that stopped her from getting results. She was training extremely hard, but still saw herself as overweight and lazy. After months of training, she had pushed herself to a point where she had become very fit. When she realised how fit she had become, even though she was still a bit overweight, her thoughts turned from lazy to healthy. As a result of this new mind set, she started to look fit and dropped her weight. The moment her self-image improved, she believed in herself and her life changed for the better.

Once upon a time there was a bunch of tiny frogs who arranged a running competition. The goal was to reach the top of a very high tower.

A big crowd had gathered around the tower to see the race and cheer on the contestants. The race began.

Honestly, no one in the crowd really believed that the tiny frogs would reach the top of the tower. You heard statements such as:

'Oh, WAY too difficult!'

'They will NEVER make it to the top.'

'Not a chance that they will succeed. The tower is too high!'

The tiny frogs began collapsing one by one ... except for those who, in a fresh tempo, were climbing higher and higher.

The crowd continued to yell, 'It is too difficult!! No one will make it!'

More tiny frogs got tired and gave up, but ONE continued. Higher and higher and higher he climbed. This one wouldn't give up!

At the end, everyone had given up climbing the tower except for the one tiny frog that, after a big effort, was the only one who reached the top!

Chapter 3 — It's All About YOU and Your Self-image

Then all of the other tiny frogs naturally wanted to know how this frog managed to do it.

A contestant asked the tiny frog how he found the strength to succeed and reach the goal. It turned out that the winner was DEAF!!

The lesson of this story is: Never listen to other people's tendencies to be negative or pessimistic because they take your most wonderful dreams and wishes away from you – the ones you have in your heart!

Always think of the power words have because everything you hear and read will affect your actions!

Therefore: ALWAYS be POSITIVE!

And above all: Be DEAF when people tell you that you cannot fulfil your dreams!

—Author Unknown

Chapter 4

– You're Only as Good as Your Attitude

"Life is 10% what happens to me and 90% how I react to it."

—**Charles Swindoll**

Attitude is the way you respond to what happens to you. Remember all sorts of things happen in life: people die, get sick, have accidents – it is called life. It is not the incident that is the problem; it is your reaction or attitude in responding to the situation that can make all the difference. Understand that the situation is neutral, and it is your attitude that can make a hell out of heaven or a heaven out of hell. When you start your body transformation, develop an attitude of consistency so you can eat clean and train, no matter what. Don't use

Chapter 4 — You're Only as Good as Your Attitude

life situations as excuses because life is full of ups and downs; but with the right attitude, you can keep exercise and healthy eating the one stable thing in your life.

Your health is directly related to your attitude. After I came home from hospital, I sunk into depression. I felt like everything I worked for was now out of reach. Had I not changed my attitude my health and state of mind would have deteriorated and I am not sure I would even be alive today. Remember, whether you think you can or you can't, you are exactly right. It is all about your attitude. Since the accident in 2001, and training for four World Fitness titles, my body has copped a bit of a pounding. I always get asked by clients, "How can you do all the training required with the injuries you have sustained?" and "Don't you feel pain when training?" Firstly, the medical diagnosis of my injuries that I live with on a day-to-day basis are:

1. Fixed patella subluxation, or permanently dislocated knee caps
2. Approximately 80% cartilage damage to both knees causing patella femoral arthritis – bone-on-bone and very creaky knees

My knees hurt all the time; and with specific training like running, stairs, or leg weights, they will swell and I will hobble around for a couple of days. My attitude was instrumental in keeping me going and I feel that I should not complain as I was hit by a train and survived. It is better to have legs that hurt than no legs at all! For that, I will be forever thankful and for Monica's weekly leg massages. The doctors all commented that being so fit before the accident and having a positive attitude in the hospital really helped me bounce back quickly.

Change Your Body with the World's Fittest Couple

The story below is a great example of what attitude to adopt when we are faced with a challenge or adversity in life.

A young woman went to her mother and told her about her life and how things were so hard for her. She did not know how she was going to make it and wanted to give up. She was tired of fighting and struggling. It seemed that as one problem was solved a new one arose.

Her mother took her to the kitchen. She filled three pots with water and placed each on a high fire. Soon the pots came to boil. In the first she placed carrots, in the second she placed eggs, and in the last she placed ground coffee beans. She let them sit and boil, without saying a word.

In about 20 minutes she turned off the burners. She fished the carrots out and placed them in a bowl. She pulled the eggs out and placed them in a bowl. Then she ladled the coffee out and placed it in a bowl.

Turning to her daughter, she asked, 'Tell me, what you see?'

'Carrots, eggs, and coffee,' she replied.

Her mother brought her closer and asked her to feel the carrots. She did and noted that they were soft. The mother then asked the daughter to take an egg and break it. After pulling off the shell, she observed the hard boiled egg. Finally, the mother asked the daughter to sip the coffee. The daughter smiled as she tasted its rich aroma.

Chapter 4 — You're Only as Good as Your Attitude

The daughter then asked 'What does it mean, mother?'

Her mother explained that each of these objects had faced the same adversity ... boiling water. Each reacted differently.

The carrot went in strong, hard, and unrelenting. However, after being subjected to the boiling water, it softened and became weak. The egg had been fragile. Its thin outer shell had protected its liquid interior, but after sitting through the boiling water its inside became hardened. The ground coffee beans were unique, however. After they were in the boiling water, they changed the water.

'Which are you?' she asked her daughter. 'When adversity and obstacles knock on your door, how do you respond? Are you a carrot, an egg, or a coffee bean?'

—Author Unknown

The brightest future will always be based on a forgotten past. You can't go forward in life until you let go of your past failures and heartaches. Yesterday is gone. Tomorrow hasn't happened. All you ever need to focus on is today. What are you going to do today that will make things easier for you tomorrow? When starting an exercise regime or stopping a destructive habit, all you should focus on is having a successful day – just take it one day at a time.

In relation to personal training, too many people focus on the end result. I always explain to them that if they were doing a long distance swim and kept on looking up at their final destination, it would stop them from getting there. All you need to do is know where you want to go and get busy getting there, and then you are assured of reaching the final destination. So in training terms, know what changes you want to make to your body and get busy each day doing what needs to be done. Keep your attitude in the present with a focus on what you would like to achieve in the future.

> *"Life at any time can become difficult; life at any time can become easy.*
>
> *It all depends upon how one adjusts oneself to life."*
>
> —Morarji Dsai

Never take life too seriously, have fun getting fit, see the funny side in trying new exercises, or making new meals. Have a laugh at yourself sometimes. We had some funny moments getting our routine ready for competitions and it was amazing how relaxed and stress free we felt after a good laugh.

In 2002, we were one week out of our first competition and practicing our fitness routine in a local gym up in Byron Bay. There is one move we do where we both wear Velcro black pants and "rip" them off each other to reveal a Tarzan and Jane outfit underneath. Anyway, we were running through the routine and a few people in the gym

Chapter 4 — You're Only as Good as Your Attitude

had gathered to watch. We got to the part where I ripped Monica's pants off and I accidentally grabbed the top part of Monica's leopard skin shorts and pulled so hard that I ripped everything off, including her underpants! Needless to say, she was left squatting down with no pants and bursting with laughter! I was laughing so hard, as were the spectators, that I forgot to hand back her pants straight away.

So, how do you want to go through life? Would you rather be a pessimist or an optimist making the most out of your life? Pessimists tend to deny problems, distance themselves from stressful events, focus on negative feelings and allow adverse situations to interfere with achieving a goal. People with a more pessimistic attitude tend to report poorer health compared to people with optimistic attitudes. Optimists, on the other hand, are able to achieve great accomplishments throughout their lives. Optimism also reduces chances of developing a disease or illness. When optimistic people become ill, they tend to recover more quickly. I am living proof of this theory.

This reminds me of an experiment that was recently conducted in Europe. Cancer patients were asked to describe how they saw their cancer as a visual image. There were two distinct visual images shared by many of the cancer patients. Group One described the cancer as a big black rat eating away at their insides. Group Two described their cancer as a bunch of mutated cells surrounded by healthy cells attacking them. The end result of the experiment was that most of Group One had died, and Group Two lived.

> *"Faith can move Mountains"*
>
> —Jesus

Change Your Body with the World's Fittest Couple

A son and his father were walking on the mountains.
Suddenly, the son falls, hurts himself, and screams,
'AAAhhhhhhhhhhh'!
To his surprise, he hears the voice repeating, somewhere in the
mountain, 'AAAhhhhhhhhhhh!'
Curious, he yells, 'Who are you?'
He receives the answer, 'Who are you?'
And then he screams to the mountain, 'I admire you!'
The voice answers, 'I admire you!'
Angered at the response, he screams, 'Coward!'
He receives the answer, 'Coward!'
He looks to his father and asks, 'What's going on?'
The father smiles and says, 'My son, pay attention.'
Again the man screams, 'You are a champion!'
The voice answers, 'You are a champion!'
The boy is surprised, but does not understand.
Then the father explains, 'People call this ECHO, but really this is LIFE. It gives you back everything you say or do. Our life is simply a reflection of our actions. If you want more love in the world, create more love in your heart. If you want more competence in your team, improve your competence. This relationship applies to everything, in all aspects of life; life will give you back everything you have given to it.'

—Author Unknown

Chapter 4 — You're Only as Good as Your Attitude

Competitive by nature, contemplating the challenge that Monica had laid down for me, and accepting what had happened to me, I now had to develop this positive attitude further – one that was strong, unwavering, and unstoppable. An affirmation I used to say to myself over and over when I was training or facing doubts was, "I can do anything."

I adopted this attitude late in my teens, and no matter what the situation, whether I had no sleep, had an exam on that morning, or sparring fight that night, I would always tell myself, "It's alright, I can do anything," and so, I did.

I did not realise the power of this affirmation until years later. When I was hit by the train and survived, my friends were not surprised. Their reaction was more like, "Yeah that sounds like Matt, taking on a train and surviving."

I would hear conversations at parties where they would be telling people about me. "He got hit by a train and then went on to win a World Fitness title." The person would reply, "How did he do that?" and my friends would just say, "He can do anything." The affirmation I would always tell myself, over and over, was now part of who I was. It's all about the attitude you develop on the inside which eventually shows on the outside.

Attitudes can even be detected in the words we use. For example, "I won't," indicates choice, whereas "I can't" indicates powerlessness. Attitudes develop when we are children. Just like changing your self-image, a pessimistic attitude won't change overnight. Start developing a more positive attitude by blocking any negative thought that enters your mind. Pay attention to your attitude in various situations to see if you have a more negative or a more pessimistic view.

The next time you are thinking or saying a negative comment, envision a large "X" marking out the negative thought. Then replace that thought, or the statement with a more positive or optimistic statement such as, "I can do anything."

Attitude is everything in life. Eliminate the negative and surround yourself with positive influences and people. Other people's attitudes will find their way into your mind, so why not fill it with positive, healthy thoughts that are yours?

Developing a "can do" attitude has literally become our greatest strength. It has been developed by getting through the tough times and pushing ourselves beyond all expectation, so that only our very best effort was acceptable as our own personal benchmark. Every area of our life has benefited from this attitude, from business to personal. When a problem arises, we almost get excited because we know that the challenge is in finding a solution. There are always options, no matter what.

> *"You may not be responsible for getting knocked down, but you are responsible for getting back up"*
>
> **—Jesse Jackson**

Chapter 4 — You're Only as Good as Your Attitude

Monica and I always focus on what we can do, not what we can't. When the problem is solved, no matter how difficult it was, the personal feeling of pride and self-satisfaction is unbelievable. It gives you much more confidence for the next challenge that comes up. Remember, sometimes it takes absolutely everything you've got.

A great example of this attitude was in 2005 when Monica was competing in the INBA Australian Championships. She had been training hard for 84 days and had a great acrobatic routine planned for the show and was fired up! Ten days before the show, I was critiquing her routine for the last time, and as she was doing a flip in the routine, she came down hard on her calf, severely tearing her calf muscle. At the time she was devastated. All her hard work and training now seemed lost, and competing in 10 days seemed near impossible.

The first thing we did was head straight to a sports physio for an accurate diagnosis. The result was a grade two tear of the calf muscle. It was serious, and the recommendation was crutches for two weeks and no activity for four weeks. When we returned home, we sat down and looked at the situation. We wrote down a list of everything that Monica could do to get herself on stage in 10 days. First of all, she loaded up on a supplement three times a day called L-Glutamine (which we will explain later in the Supplement Section). This is an awesome supplement for repairing muscle tissue and replenishing the body after injury trauma.

Monica's greatest strength in fitness competitions was undoubtedly her explosive acrobatic moves and aerial cartwheels. This was not possible with a torn calf, so the routine had to be changed. We worked out all the moves she could still do and came up with a routine where, for the majority of the 90 seconds, she was on her hands. We decided to put a wooden step platform in the routine so that she actually walked out from behind the curtains on her hands and then continued to walk up the stairs of the platform on her hands. She then flipped onto her backside and went straight into upper body strength moves on top of the platform before walking down the other side still on her hands, completing her routine using many non weight-bearing moves.

Rather than pull out of the competition due to injury, Monica decided to face the challenge head-on and go for it!

After the routine, the crowd was mesmerized. It was a completely different routine than they were used to seeing, and it worked in her favour, big time, without anyone even knowing about the injury. Monica went on the win the competition, and to this day, some people still comment that it is the best routine she has ever done.

The happiest of people don't necessarily have the best of everything; they just make the most of everything that comes along their way.

—**Author unknown**

Chapter 5
– Setting Goals

"Plan for the future because that is where you are going to spend the rest of your life."

—**Mark Twain**, 1835 - 1910

Now that you've determined your source of motivation for change and the importance of a positive self-image and a strong unwavering attitude, you need to make a plan to achieve your goals. The first thing you need to do is realise that, no matter who you are, every journey has a starting point, and it's going to be different for each person. Some people are naturally more fit than others. Don't let this deter you. With motivation, discipline, and focus, you can achieve the highest level of fitness.

Two weeks out of the hospital after my accident, Monica challenged me to compete with her in a World Fitness Competition in Germany. The competition was in 18 months. How could I take part in a competition in such a short time? Doctors had told me to find a new career and that I would more than likely never run again. Someone else's opinion of you does not have to become your reality. I pushed their opinions out of my mind and set my mind in motion for a journey of healing and full recovery. By setting goals and striving to meet them, I was able to defy the doctors. My first goal was to learn how to walk again. With little to no cartilage in my knees and stretched ligaments, this seemed impossible. I didn't think about any of that and focused on my goal. I was going to compete with Monica, no matter what.

By staying motivated and dedicated to my goal, I went from bending to standing, balancing to walking, and eventually cycling. I accredit my success, in part, to effective goal setting. You need to set effective goals to reach your highest level of fitness.

When you set a goal, try to remember the following:

- Make all of your statements very positive and put them in the present tense.
- Precision is important. To enable you to measure your accomplishments, include dates, times, and amounts. This lets you know if you're exact.
- Give each goal a priority. By doing this, you won't feel too overwhelmed by your goals. This also helps you to direct your attention to the most important goals.
- Write your goals down.

- Don't listen to anyone other than yourself. People will always try to tell you that your goals are just dreams and you will never achieve them. Eliminate that negative energy from your life. Repeat to yourself every day that whatever you put your mind to do, you can and will accomplish.
- A goal is a dream with a deadline

Set yourself a fitness goal today! Whether it is entering a competition 6 to 12 months away or losing weight, you must write it down on a large piece of paper and put it up where you will see it every day. We laminate our goals and put them up in our shower. Put up positive affirmations around your home to keep you on track with your fitness goal.

Our favourite affirmations and their locations at home and work are:

- Stay dedicated (fridge, exercise bike)
- Confidence wins (mirror)
- Never ever give up (office)
- Stop. Think. Evaluate. Proceed (fridge)
- Nothing tastes as good as fit feels (pantry)
- Give 100% in training and diet – anything less is a waste of time and energy (next to bed)

They really help to keep us on track, especially on those cold mornings when we are too tired or when we felt like eating something unhealthy!

Thinking a Goal Through

When you think about how to achieve your goals, think about what can help you to focus and lead to achievement. Ask yourself the following questions:

- What skills do I need to achieve this?
- What information and knowledge do I need?
- What help, assistance, or collaboration do I need?
- What resources do I need or have?
- What can keep me from making progress?
- Am I making assumptions? What are they?
- Is there a better way of achieving this goal?

When I thought about all of this, I already had all the information. I had studied exercise science and knew what to do: I started to write down my action plan.

I had a timeline of 18 months, and I set small goals along the way. In the first four weeks, I wanted to be riding my bike. To achieve this goal, I went to three physiotherapy sessions a week and did all my balance and stabilization drills. In week four, there I was, cycling up the street just as Monica drove past in her car with a fixed stare on me, nearly driving into a fence! At the time, I still had a plaster cast on my leg, another on my arm, and no teeth – but, at least I had made my goal!

The next goal was jogging in week eight. To achieve this, I had to cut my cast off my leg in week six, throw away the crutches, and begin moving faster. Sure enough, by week eight I was jogging. It may have been slower than a Cliff Young shuffle, but I was jogging! For those of

Chapter 5 — Setting Goals

you who don't know what the "Cliff Young shuffle" is, here is a quick summary:

Australia used to host a 600 kilometre foot race from Sydney to Melbourne from 1983 to 1991. In the inaugural race, a 61 year old bush farmer that use to round up cows in his gumboots for training– Cliff Young fell well behind the professional long distance runners. However, as all of the other runners turned in for the night, Cliff Young kept on shuffling until he was in the lead by midnight. Young only slept for 2 hours and at 2am, was back on the road again. When the other runners started again on day two – "Cliffy Young" was 40 kilometres in front. 10 pairs of runners later, virtually no sleep, a shoulder injury and massive blisters, Cliff Young shuffled in to Melbourne at midnight on day 6 – well in front, becoming a great Australian hero.

From then on, sleeping was not an option if you wanted to win the Melbourne to Sydney Ultra Marathon. To win that race, you had to run all night and all day at the "Cliff Young shuffle pace".

So, I just kept referring to the goals on my timeline and doing everything I could to make it happen. It didn't always go to plan, and I definitely had a lot of obstacles and challenges along the way, but I didn't give up.

Visualising Your Goals

Believing that you can hurdle barriers and achieve your goals is your ticket to success. One of the most powerful tools for accomplishing goals is visualisation.

This easy technique involves imagining the accomplishment of your goals. By visualising your goals, you are training your mind to achieve your goals.

Unfortunately, most people unconsciously use visualisation when they worry about things. They make themselves sick by dwelling on the negative things in life – over things that will never even happen. You attract what you think about. If you visualise negative thoughts then your life will be filled with stress and adversity. You've lost that time forever. That was time you could have spent thinking about something more positive and productive. You can train yourself to dwell in possibility, thinking about positive things, like your goals.

Power of Visualisation

Dr. Denis Waitley, author of *The Psychology of Winning,* the trainer of the astronauts in the Apollo space program, and possibly one of the greatest American lecturers on high performance human achievement, shows the amazing effects of visualisation in this following story. He took the visualisation process from his Apollo program and instituted it during the 1980's and 1990's into the Olympic program. It was called Visual Motor Rehearsal, and he outlines it below:

"When you visualise then you materialize. Here's an interesting thing about the mind: we took Olympic athletes and had them run their event only in their mind, and then hooked them up to sophisticated biofeedback equipment. Incredibly, the same muscles fired in the same sequence when they were running the race in their mind as when they were running it on the track. How could this be? Because the mind can't distinguish whether you're really doing it or whether it's just a practice. If you have been there in the mind you'll go there in the body."

Visualising every detail of every step in a given activity creates, modifies, and strengthens brain pathways that are important in coordinating your muscles for the visualised activity. This prepares you to perform the activity itself. The technique is useful in many areas of life – from avoiding the anxieties of everyday life to performing well during competition. This is a powerful tool in training for fitness. Visualisation takes little effort or time to do, but it's the best and most overlooked component to quickly fulfilling your achievements.

Every day, I would picture myself onstage: ripped, strong, and invincible. I just kept on thinking I was going to get there no matter what. Monica always made sure she had done everything she could do in her 84 day preparation to win her fitness competitions. In her fitness career she came in first place, 13 out of 17 competitions that she competed in. Monica had "tunnel vision" for 84 days and would have her acrobatic routines developed very early on so she could perfect them before competition. This enabled her to walk on that stage with confidence that she was the best, and it showed every time. We would visualise together on the plane to Europe, what it would feel like to hold the trophy and execute a perfect routine. This gave us unbelievable confidence and excitement. We had no room for self-doubt.

Now, I don't consider myself to be an artist, but I do like drawing cartoons when I am thinking or visualising.

On the plane to Germany for the 2002 Fitness Universe, while I was visualising doing the routine on stage, I started drawing a little cartoon. Below is the actual cartoon I drew on the plane while we were visualising . . . and of course it came true!

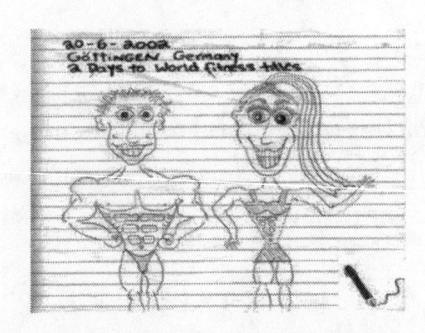

Take yourself deep into the emotion as if you are accomplishing your goal and it will energize you. Imagine the new clothes you will buy, the energy you will have, the holiday you will go on, running through the finish line of a fun run, receiving the trophy at the competition you have entered or completing your first marathon. It is really possible to change your thoughts and therefore your body. All great athletes know that the subconscious mind is the most powerful advantage they have. It is your brain. Get it working for you and you will have an amazing life.

Spend a few moments right now visualising. Read the following steps, then close your eyes and let your body relax.

- Identify the goal you want to visualise, for example, running a fun run, being in a size 10 or 12 outfit, or a smart suit.
- Eliminate all distractions – turn off your phones, televisions, and radios.
- Free your mind of negative thoughts.
- Create a picture in your mind of the place – the sights, sounds, and smells. Imagine a perfect day, great weather. Picture yourself with your favourite running buddies, talking and laughing.

Now, visualise yourself starting on your way, passing the spectators, and setting off to run the whole course. Visualise yourself going shopping for that new outfit. Visualise the feeling of wearing any clothes you like and walking confidently down the street.

- Take a moment to feel the pleasure and excitement of achieving this goal.
- Then visualise yourself crossing the finish line, or going to a party or function feeling great, both physically and emotionally.

Your mind's ability to feel and experience your goals as already having been achieved will embed the emotion of success into your body and into your subconscious mind. Your subconscious mind doesn't know the difference between a picture in your mind's eye and what is real. You will begin to find yourself getting very emotional and experiencing true joy just thinking about your goal.

Once you can *see* the sort of life you want, your mind will lead you in the right direction to achieve it. The most important thing is to trust this process and try it every day; you only need a few minutes. Unless you believe in it, it won't work for you. Try it for just three months. You'll see the results for yourself.

Another way to create lasting change in your life is by writing down a vision of what your ideal life would be like. To change your life from where you are today to something better, you must first be able to *see* what sort of life you would like to have. Monica writes down her vision once a year. Here are a couple of paragraphs from her ideal life vision that she wrote in 2007:

Change Your Body with the World's Fittest Couple

"I get up when my body is ready, always starting the day with a run along the river with my dog Ralph, then a weights workout, and yoga. Matt and I travel the world teaching people how to change their bodies and lives. We love seeing the transformation take place and watching as both children and adults start making healthy habits to prolong their life. It is our mission to help rid the world of obesity through our best selling books. We train, work, and live together like peas in a pod! We love walking along the beaches of the world and exploring new destinations in our time off. Our life is full of love, adventure, travel, friends, family, laughter, and children."

How was that for a life vision? Sounds pretty good doesn't it? Now it may seem pretty far-fetched or pie in the sky to you, but write down whatever excites you. No one else has to see it, or even believe it . . . only you. Every vision we have ever written down has come true! My vision contains the three words "best selling authors", so let's wait and see on that one!

"Get excited and enthusiastic about your own dream. This excitement is like a forest fire – you can smell it, taste it, and see it from a mile away."

—**Denis Waitley**

Chapter 5 — Setting Goals

Now it is your turn to write one. Do it and feel the excitement you get from creating your ideal life. Then, once it is written, laminate it and put it beside your bed to read before you sleep each night, or for times when you are not charged about life.

Remember that goals give your life meaning. Goals increase your confidence. Goals boost your level of motivation. Goals give you a sense of purpose. You become what you think about most of the time. Know exactly what it is you want. Determine the price you will have to pay to achieve your goals, and then get busy!

"Forget past mistakes. Forget failures. Forget everything except what you're going to do now, and do it".

—William Durant

Chapter 6

– Discipline

If today you don't eat chocolate – you will make no difference to the shape of your body. If you don't eat chocolate again tomorrow there will still be no change. But if you do the same thing every day for a couple of months, you'll see an impressive alteration.

No matter how much we desire transformation, we often find the only way to attain it is to make effort, with commitment, over time. We are surrounded by examples of what can be accomplished with patience and dedication.

Stay focused, create healthy habits, and be consistent every day!

Chapter 6 — Discipline

Discipline, commitment, and consistency helped me through my trials and struggles. These are the cornerstones in any fitness lifestyle. You may be able to exercise and begin to feel healthy, but this will be short-lived, and fade away over time if you don't actively focus on these three areas.

At times, especially during rehabilitation, I experienced pain to the point where I would want to stop. The most painful time was at the osteopath where Josh, my osteopath, is no stranger to inflicting pain on his clients – for the greater good of course. One of the worst injuries I sustained was a 30 centimetre cut on my inner left thigh down past my knee to my calf, where I had been impaled to the bone by my bike. So, in these treatments, I would receive a scar tissue massage to break up the purple chunky scar in order to gain mobility. Josh would achieve this by pinching the skin in his fingers and pulling. This was absolutely excruciating, but I would just keep telling myself, "Ten more seconds," then I'd have a short break, then again "10 more seconds."

If I did not have a goal of increasing my mobility so I could achieve a slow jog at the eight week mark, there is no way I would have returned to Josh for another torture session. It amazes me how quickly the brain forgets pain. I often ask my clients this question, "Tell me, what was the hardest, most painful session you have ever done with me?" This question always draws a blank. What might be extremely painful at the time becomes a forgotten memory. Our ability to forget pain serves us well in life; otherwise, there would be a lot of families out there with only one child!

> *"True enjoyment comes from activity*
> *of the mind and exercise of the body;*
> *the two are always united".*
>
> —**Alexander von Humboldt**, 1769 - 1859

Discipline is about following through, taking the challenge one day at a time, getting it done in parts, and sticking to it no matter what. It makes no difference where you start as long as each day you have the discipline to improve by at least 1%. If you have this as your philosophy, plus the discipline to carry it out, then think about how much you would improve after a year. For example, with many clients who hate running, we start them off on our run challenge, which is just 20 seconds to start. Then, every day, they have to add another 20 seconds. The challenge is to see how long they can keep this daily 20 second add-on. We have had several clients achieve the daily twenty second add on for a year and this resulted in a very impressive two hours of running! This training technique works really well, for if they miss three days of training, they have to add one minute. The longer they leave it, the harder it gets because they have not conditioned their bodies. If they run each day, then the small accomplishments are more achievable.

A challenge that I did in 2005 with my brother and five mates was the New Year's Eve Push-Up Challenge. We all put $100 into the kitty with a pact: 100 push-ups on January 1 and add one push-up each day until the end of the year. We are all extremely competitive, so no one intentionally pulled out. By the end of the year, only two out of the seven guys completed the challenge – my brother Simm and my mate Mick. The total number of push-ups on December 31 was 465. The total amount of push-ups done over the year was 103,000. Now you

Chapter 6 — Discipline

are probably thinking, "Well you're pretty competitive, why didn't you win?" It goes like this . . . I returned home after a wedding and went in the lounge room to do my 290 push-ups. After completing my first set of 100, I lay on the couch for a rest and fell asleep, waking at 2:00 a.m! Because of the rule stipulations, I was out. Little challenges like these are great ways to develop discipline. At the same time they increase your health and fitness.

Discipline enables you to persevere in whatever you choose to do. You will be able to withstand any hardships, struggles, or difficulties, whether they are physical or emotional. Through discipline, you will become conscious of your subconscious impulses and gain the ability to dismiss them if they aren't for your own good. Soon after you've developed discipline, you will feel powerful and in command of your surroundings and environment, which will lead you to a life filled with health and fitness.

> *"The greatest discovery of my generation is that human beings can alter their lives by altering their attitudes of mind."*
>
> **—William James**

On occasion, do you ever want to go to the gym knowing how good it is for your health and how great you feel afterward, yet, you feel too lazy, and would rather stay at home and watch TV instead? You might also be aware of the fact that you need to change your eating habits or stop drinking; yet you don't have the discipline to change these habits.

Does this sound familiar? How many times have you told yourself, "I wish I had willpower and self-discipline?" How many times have you started to do something, only to quit after a short while? Each one of us has had experiences like these.

We all have some bad habits, whether they are overeating, laziness, smoking, drinking, or procrastination. Discipline with no excuses is the key to overcoming these habits. When Monica and I train clients, we have a no excuse policy. The moment we see a client start to make too many excuses, we stop working with them.

One of our first clients, Jerome, had no discipline when it came to exercising alone. He just would not do it. He understood the importance of exercise as it related to his health, for he liked to live a fun and fast lifestyle. He was submerged in the hospitality industry where he worked hard and played even harder. When he asked me to train him four times a week, I specifically told him that I would, without a doubt, stop the training if his lifestyle became an excuse. Jerome would go out at night and party until 3:00 a.m. He didn't let this hinder his desire to be fit; he would change into his workout clothes as soon as he got home and sleep in them so he would be ready at 6:00 a.m. when I picked him up.

By understanding the importance of exercise and his own personality, he created a successful plan that worked for him. It is clearly not the best example of a balanced or healthy lifestyle, but no matter how late a night or how many drinks, he was up and ready to go the next morning. Over a four-year period, he hardly missed a session. This type of discipline makes a great difference in life. It brings inner strength and a life balanced between the mind and body.

Chapter 6 — Discipline

Developing Willpower and Self-discipline

One way to develop and improve your discipline is to do something that you don't like. Your mind and body won't like this, but don't stop. Let me explain. By doing things you hate doing, you overcome your subconscious resistances, train your inner powers, and gain inner strength. Just like your muscles get stronger by resisting the power of the weights, so does your mind. In personal training, we see this all the time.

One particular morning, I was training a young and vocal girl called Grace. We were doing stair runs and plyometric conditioning exercises – in other words: pain. She hated it. Trainers know that when people are in pain, they will do or say anything to get out of the exercise. Grace thought she would start with a bit of personal abuse; "I am not doing it you ugly #@!#." My reply was, "That's great Grace, now give me five more."

Then she really started. "I hate your guts and I am never doing this again, you #@!#." My reply was, "No worries, but we are not leaving here this morning until you are finished."

So for the rest of the session, amidst the abuse, Grace did the work and hated every second. I was not ready for what she said at the end of the session: "Matt, that was a great session, can we do that again next week?" What the #@!#! Grace might have hated the session, but she felt a real sense of accomplishment, self-satisfaction, and an endorphin buzz at the end.

Through the sport of fitness, we have competed around the world, and the biggest element to our training is discipline. We use discipline to train and exercise every day as well as eat healthy, and to give our bodies what they need.

Fitness is probably one of the most disciplined sports on the planet because you have to train and diet – HARD. People these days lack the discipline to say NO to themselves about unhealthy foods, and say YES to themselves about exercise.

Shake It Off and Step Up

A parable is told of a farmer who owned an old mule. The mule fell into the farmer's well. The farmer heard the mule braying or whatever mules do when they fall into wells. After carefully assessing the situation, the farmer sympathized with the mule but decided that neither the mule nor the well was worth the trouble of saving. Instead, he called his neighbors together and told them what had happened, and enlisted them to help haul dirt to bury the old mule in the well and put him out of his misery.

Initially, the old mule was hysterical! But, as the farmer and his neighbors continued shoveling and the dirt hit his back, a thought struck him. It suddenly dawned on him that every time a shovel load of dirt landed on his back, HE COULD SHAKE IT OFF AND STEP UP! This he did, blow after blow.

"Shake it off and step up ... shake it off and step up ... shake it off and step up!" he repeated to encourage himself. No matter how painful the blows or distressing the situation seemed, the old mule fought panic and just kept right on SHAKING IT OFF AND STEPPING UP!

Chapter 6 — Discipline

You're right! It wasn't long before the old mule, battered and exhausted, STEPPED TRIUMPHANTLY OVER THE WALL OF THAT WELL! What seemed like was sure to bury him actually blessed him ... all because of the manner in which he handled his adversity.

THAT'S LIFE! If we face our problems and respond to them positively, and refuse to give in to panic, bitterness, or self-pity, THE ADVERSITIES THAT COME ALONG TO BURY US USUALLY HAVE WITHIN THEM THE POTENTIAL TO BENEFIT AND BLESS US!

Remember that FORGIVENESS, FAITH, BEING GRATEFUL FOR WHAT YOU HAVE, and HOPE are excellent ways to SHAKE IT OFF AND STEP UP out of the wells in which we find ourselves!

—**Author Unknown**

Try the following exercises to improve your discipline:

- Add an extra 10 minutes onto everything you do. You'll be surprised at the things you will find out or even accomplish in a day!
    - 10 more minutes exercising will give you a better body.
    - 10 more minutes studying and you might finally understand the answer or formula.
    - 10 more minutes sleeping will do your body and mind wonders.

- 10 more minutes surfing the Internet and you might find an awesome site you didn't even know existed.
- 10 more minutes to eat your meals – eating slowly is much better for your digestive system, and you will find yourself eating less because you feel full sooner.

- There is laundry that needs washing, and you postpone washing it until later. Get up and wash it now. Do not let your laziness overcome you. When you know you are developing your self-discipline, and if you are convinced of its importance, it will be easier for you to do whatever you have to do.
- You know you need to go to the gym, but instead you sit and do nothing or watch a movie. Get up and walk, run, or do some other physical exercise.
- Do you like your coffee with sugar? Then for a whole week decide to drink it without sugar.
- You like to drink three cans of soda each day? For a week drink only one can and two bottles of water.
- You have a desire to eat a piece of chocolate? Instead eat a piece of fruit.

One little discipline training trick I adopted in my life was that when my intuition or subconscious was telling me to do something constructive or positive, then I would do it immediately. If someone suggested I try something, or do a task that might help with my overall goal, I would say yes and give it a go. It came down to a philosophy I call THINK IT, DO IT.

Overcome your laziness and convince yourself of the importance of what is to be done. Convince your mind that you gain inner strength when you act and do things, in spite of your inner

Chapter 6 — Discipline

resistance. You can't achieve any goal without discipline. You have to exercise and train even when you don't feel like it.

Have you ever found yourself staring at an untidy room, wondering just how to begin the process of putting it in order? If so, you'll know that ultimately it doesn't make much difference. You can start in a corner or the middle of the floor. The important thing is to roll up your sleeves and start somewhere. As long as you stand looking at the untidy room, the job looks too hard. The moment you get to grips with it, it will become easy.

I love listening to motivational CD's when I am driving. I find it inspires me to reach my goals, and I love listening to great mentors speak their pearls of wisdom. One of my personal favourites is Jim Rohn. The following is from a Jim Rohn CD I heard in the car:

"Some people don't do well simply because they don't feel well. Some people take better care of their pets than they do of themselves. Their animals can run like the wind and they can barely make it up a flight of stairs.

"Make sure the outside of you is a good reflection of the inside of you. Treat your body like a temple, not a woodshed. The mind and the body work together. Your body needs to be a good support system for the mind and spirit. If you take good care of it, your body takes you wherever you want to go, with the power, strength, energy and vitality you will need to get there."

Remember there are two pains in life, the Pain of Regret and the Pain of Discipline. One weighs tons while the other weighs grams. Don't let the lack of discipline keep you from living an amazing and energy-filled life.

> *"Tomorrow is the most important
> thing in life.
> It comes into us at midnight very clean.
> It's perfect when it arrives and it puts
> itself in our hands.
> It hopes we've learned something
> from yesterday."*
>
> —**John Wayne**, 1907 - 1979

Chapter 7

– Commitment

> *"A man too busy to take care of his health is like a mechanic too busy to take care of his tools."*
>
> **—Spanish Proverb**

The most important single factor in your success is commitment. You see, commitment ignites action, and to commit is to pledge yourself to a healthy eating and physical training regime.

Two important conditions for commitment are:

- A strong belief system.
- Surround yourself with people whose beliefs are the same as yours.

Your commitment to a healthy lifestyle depends on how strongly you believe in its importance and how faithfully you carry out your actions, such as healthy eating and exercising. I have trained thousands of clients. It is neither the strongest nor the fittest clients who have impressed me the most with their results. It is the clients that keep on turning up no matter what, that always seem to be in the background, just getting on with it. Too many people start, but don't finish. Those individuals that made a personal commitment to become fit and healthy eventually got some astounding, life-changing results.

Fit and healthy individuals that are committed to their health, possess a strong sense of personal integrity, self-confidence, and happiness. Exercise and healthy eating becomes a wonderful habit that instils a sense of self worth and confidence in people. Continual self-improvement has no finish line. There are no limitations to what you can do in this life. Being committed to a healthy eating and exercise regime goes hand-in-hand with your success and happiness at work and at home.

There can be no courage when there is no confidence. Half the battle is in the conviction that you can accomplish what you want. Confidence doesn't come out of nowhere; it's the result of work and dedication. With practice, you will come to a point of competence. You will find yourself accomplishing things gracefully and confidently. It's then that things will become easier and you will start to achieve your dreams. When you are prepared, you are able to feel more confident.

Chapter 7 — Commitment

When we are backstage on competition day and right up to the awards ceremony, there is one affirmation that we say to ourselves and each other at least a hundred times that day: CONFIDENCE WINS. That's our total focus. We are not focused on remembering the routine or looking in the mirror wishing we had trained our legs a little more. On that day, all the hard work is done and nothing else matters except confidence on stage.

The combination of a strong, positive commitment to yourself and to a set of principles serves as a foundation to effectively maintain a healthy lifestyle for the mind and body. Besides feeling great, commitments to health can also target specific results. Given the large number of demands placed on all of us, it is important to concentrate on achieving the most important goals and objectives. Commitment to results is largely determined by how clear priorities are, what actions get rewarded, and what risks are being taken to improve your quality of life.

Once you have made a commitment to yourself to achieve your goal, there is one more promise you have to make to yourself and keep, no matter what. Promise that regardless of what happens, you will never, ever give up.

My favourite cartoon of all time is the picture of the frog and the stork. I have this picture at home and in my office. I absolutely love its powerful message.

NEVER EVER EVER GIVE UP

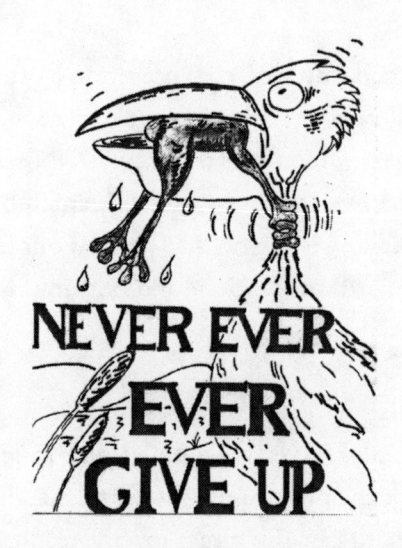

Redrawn, original cartoonist unknown

If you come off the rails, BIG DEAL, WHO CARES? You have blown nothing; get back on track the next day. It happens, learn from it, make a plan so it doesn't happen again, and then dump it. Don't use it as an excuse to stop, like, "Oh well, I've blown it now, I'm never going to lose weight", and go back to your old habits. Remember, it is what you do 90% of the time that counts, the other 10% makes no difference.

"At some stage you will experience a plateau – as if everything had stopped. This is a hard point in the journey. Know that once the process has started it doesn't stop; it only appears to stop from where you are looking."

—**Ram Dass**

The other important condition for commitment is surrounding yourself with people whose beliefs are the same as yours. Your surrounding environment is crucial to your success. You might have all the best intentions in the world to eat clean and exercise every day. But, if you go home and everyone is eating fast food and drinking beer every night, or your workplace is surrounded with biscuits and sweet bowls, or your best friend lives an unhealthy lifestyle, then the temptation and frustration will eventually become too much. You had better have the discipline and commitment of a Tibetan monk because – believe me, no one is that strong.

As I mentioned earlier, my WHY has always been triggered by my competitive spirit. But the biggest reason for my success in fitness competitions has been my environment. At home, I live on what I call "Planet Monica", where my surrounding environment is filled with energy, healthy food, and water. My brother, Simm came to live with us in 2003. At the time, he was a drummer in a rock band, manager of a night club, and lived a fast lifestyle, food included. Because he was living on "Planet Monica", he had no choice but to eat the food we prepared and do the activities that we did. In four months, he lost 10 kilograms and became the fittest that he had ever been, just by living with us and adopting the healthy habits that we follow each day. Today Simm is one of the most disciplined and fittest people we know.

Practising Commitment

Effectively demonstrating commitment to your health is never easy. The truth is that demonstrating commitment is hard work. Wavering commitment is the easy way out. The only way to achieve results through commitment is through determination and persistence. Genuine commitment stands the test of time.

Each day, commitment is demonstrated by combining two actions:

- Support. This develops a commitment in the minds of those around you. By having a strong sense of commitment, you can lead others to a healthy lifestyle by example. Support means concentrating on the things that add value, spotlighting exercise programs that work, and rewarding others who are focusing on what is important. A crucial aspect of true support is standing up to those who would undermine commitment, those whose words or actions show disrespect.

- Improvement. Improving stretches your commitment to an even higher level. Commitment means a willingness to search for a better way and learn from the process. It focuses on eliminating complacency, confronting programs that aren't working, and providing incentives for improvement. The spirit of improving is embedded in challenging your current expectations and ultimately taking the risk to make changes. These changes are based more on optimism in the future than dissatisfaction with the past.

When Commitment is Most Difficult

Commitment is most difficult and most readily proven during times of strife. How a person wards off the temptation to take a break from exercising, or falls into the line of thought that "Just one bite won't kill me" most clearly demonstrates their basic belief about healthy living.

It is easiest to compromise your commitment to good health during times such as holidays or vacations. The real test comes when you can hold the line against the easy route of compromise. Commitment is a two-way street. You only get it if you are willing to give it.

Chapter 7 — Commitment

During the final 84 days of strict eating and training preparation in our first year of fitness competitions, we had three weddings and an awards night to attend. On all of these occasions, the food was incredible, but we didn't have a single bite. Everyone around us was eating rich foods and drinking alcohol. Not going to these events was not an option for us. Just because we cannot indulge does not mean we cannot socialize and celebrate with friends. To stick to our commitment, we just had to be prepared with a plan. Weeks earlier, Monica had organized special low sodium clean meals at the weddings, and we took our own food to the awards night. When you are surrounded by your best friends, alcohol, and fresh chocolate cake, it can be extremely hard not to indulge. The next day, though, when you get up, the temptation is gone. The feeling of empowerment and self-achievement that flows over you from sticking to your personal commitment feels awesome.

Keep yourself on track by following the "Shower Power" statements below; a great tip that we picked up from John McGrath's book, *YOU Inc.*

Shower Power

Ask yourself these questions every day in the shower to keep on track (type these up and laminate them and paste on shower wall):

- What are the things in my life that make me happy?
- What will I do to make a difference in someone's life today?
- How will I exercise today to increase my energy and make me stronger?
- What food will I eat today to give me energy and cleanse me?

Chapter 8

– Consistency and Creating Healthy Habits

"We are what we repeatedly do. Excellence, therefore, is not an act but a habit."

—**Aristotle**

Consistency is a crucial step in your journey to fitness and wellness. About 90% of success is just showing up. If you don't show up to the gym, jogging trail, or any place else that you train and exercise, then you won't get any better. If you don't make a workout, you not only don't take a step forward, you take one backward. Once you have made a plan to follow the right exercise and diet program prescribed for you, all you need to do is stick to it. There is no need to do any more or any less. Follow your program! If you are consistent, the results will come!

Chapter 8 — Consistency and Creating Healthy Habits

Be prepared to train. If you fail to prepare, you are preparing for failure. To be consistent, you must commit to your best effort, have a vision for daily progress, and focus time and energy on things that get you closer to your goal. The fittest people are consistent in their approach to all parts of their training – every day!

No one is going to care more about your training and development than you. You have to work as hard as you can to get the most out of your program. You will have times when you have days off from training and light intensity days. This is okay, as long as you continue to be consistent in your workout program. Besides, you'll need these days; recovery is critical. However, when it is time to work, you have to go hard! Hard work combined with consistency can accomplish anything. When it comes to training I always say "Get in, Give it your best and Get out!

We constantly tell clients that if they follow our program, commit to it and do it consistently then they will get results. If they nearly do it all, or almost do it, then they will nearly get results. We see people in other gyms all the time that work out harder than we do. They train with great intensity and then disappear for two weeks. Hence, they don't change; they just stay the same. Some people do the same program or class for weeks on end with no results. The body needs to be shocked every six to eight weeks and given a different program, or it will not achieve results. We will cover this in greater detail in the "Move It to Lose It" section.

When changing the shape of your body, consistency beats intensity. However, if you add consistency and intensity together, you can achieve any amount of success. Finish whatever you begin, and experience the triumph of completion.

> *"Finish every day and be done with it. You have done what you could. Some blunders and absurdities no doubt crept in; forget them as soon as you can.*
>
> *Tomorrow is a new day; begin it well and serenely and with too high a spirit to be cumbered with your old nonsense. This day is all that is good and fair.*
>
> *It is too dear, with its hopes and invitations, to waste a moment on yesterdays."*
>
> **—Ralph Waldo Emerson**, 1803 - 1882

Consistency means sticking to your plan when you are exhausted, stressed, or have been working all day. It doesn't matter. You just need to get the job done. Monica is one of the most consistent women I have ever met when it comes to exercise and eating healthy. She will exercise 365 days and eat clean 360, whereas I definitely have an off season.

Chapter 8 — Consistency and Creating Healthy Habits

A perfect example of how consistent and strict Monica is with our food preparation was during our 84 day competition diet in 2002, while we were getting ready for our first Fitness Universe Competition. We always allow ourselves a take-away roast chicken once a week, instead of cooking our own chicken. We have it with a large salad or steamed vegetables. When I pull apart a roast chicken, I love to lick my fingers at the end; it is something I have done since I was young! So here I am, getting dinner ready, and out of habit, I went to lick my fingers after pulling apart the chicken. Out of nowhere, Monica sprang from behind me and grabbed my hand just as I was opening my mouth! She said, "Don't even think about it you finger licker! Your fingers are covered with seasoning and fat."

I was crushed and didn't realise what I was doing. It was just one of those habits. I guess I have always been a finger licker! I washed my hands instead. She even went so far as to place the roast chicken pieces on a serviette and press all the excess oil out!

"Motivation is what gets you started.
Habit is what keeps you going."

—Jim Ryun

Chapter 9
– Overcoming Obstacles

"If you're trying to achieve, there will be roadblocks. I've had them; everybody has had them. But obstacles don't have to stop you. If you run into a wall, don't turn around and give up. Figure out how to climb it, go through it, or work around it."

—**Michael Jordan**

Do you give up after you make a mistake? Mistakes are okay. No one is perfect. The only unforgivable mistake is the one you don't learn from. Don't look at mistakes as setbacks or obstacles; look at mistakes as learning tools instead.

Chapter 9 — Overcoming Obstacles

Obstacles don't matter much to the end result if you keep going forward. If you wish to enjoy the world's pleasures you must also endure its pains. You will find that most things are difficult before they are easy. The story of the giraffe learning to walk is a great example of this.

The Giraffe Story

Bringing a giraffe into the world is a tall order. A baby giraffe falls 10 feet from its mother's womb and usually lands on its back. Within seconds, it rolls over and tucks its legs under its body. From this position it considers the world for the first time and shakes off the last vestiges of birthing fluid from its eyes and ears. Then the mother giraffe rudely introduces its offspring to the reality of life.

" The mother giraffe lowers her head long enough to take a quick look. Then she positions herself directly over her calf. She waits for about a minute, and then she does the most unreasonable thing. She swings her long, pendulous leg outward and kicks her baby, so that it is sent sprawling head over heels.

When it doesn't get up, the violent process is repeated over and over again. The struggle to rise is momentous. As the calf grows tired, the mother kicks it again to stimulate its efforts. Finally, the calf stands for the first time on its wobbly legs.

Then the mother giraffe does the most remarkable thing. She kicks it off its feet again. Why? She wants it to remember how it got up. In the wild, baby giraffes must be able to get up as quickly as possible to stay with the herd, where there is safety. Lions, hyenas, leopards, and wild hunting dogs all enjoy young giraffes, and they'd get them, too, if the mother didn't teach her calf to get up quickly and get with it."

—**Craig B. Larson**,
Illustrations for Preaching and Teaching, Leadership Journal
Gary Richmond, A View from the Zoo

Nothing in life is to be feared, it is only to be understood. When you face the things that scare you, you open the door to freedom and success. Most obstacles will melt away if you stand up to them rather than giving in or procrastinating about dealing with them.

Obstacles may be the distracting, negative self-talk that we call the "mind monkeys" that play games inside your head, such as, "I'll start exercising tomorrow," or "I'll eat this chocolate now and start my diet tomorrow." People say this to themselves their whole life! Defeat the mind monkeys. Stand up strong to them and they will disappear, guaranteed. When I was training, every time those annoying mind monkeys put an image in my head of me standing on stage in my little red budgie smugglers (brief Australian underwear), skinny chicken legs with the crowd pointing and laughing, I would drop down immediately and pump out 100 push-ups. I have done push ups just about everywhere, even aisle three of the supermarket! This action soon shut up the mind monkeys and by the second Fitness Universe competition in Germany, that fear had completely gone.

Don't be afraid to take the steps you need to make positive changes in your life. To fight fears you must act. Fears grow in magnitude when you do nothing. The greater the obstacle, the greater the satisfaction in overcoming the obstacle. Before you begin, know that sacrifice is going to be part of the package.

Chapter 9 — Overcoming Obstacles

Sooner or later, you'll experience a crisis in your life. How you deal with it will determine your future happiness and success. When a crisis comes your way, don't react straight away, let it sit in your mind and give it meaning. There is a reason this crisis has come into your life. Spend some time figuring out the reason why you have been challenged with this crisis. Personal growth is the process of responding positively to change. A precious stone cannot be polished without friction!

> *"Press on. Obstacles are seldom the same size tomorrow as they are today."*
>
> **—Robert H. Schuller**

We competed in our very first fitness pair's competition in Queensland in 2002. It was a qualifier for the 2002 Fitness Universe. Monica had been competing for four years and she already had experience in dieting, making up the fitness routines, and getting ready on the day. This preparation included tanning the whole body for stage appearance. The first thing I was told to do was to have a shower and shave off all my body hair in preparation for the tanning colour we had to apply. I was a little nervous with my first competition and we were also running very late, so I rushed through the process and I cut my shin open with the shaver trying to shave my legs. There was blood everywhere. We held a towel to it, but it was still bleeding after 20 minutes. So we raced to the chemist and got it patched up. I had to apply the stage tanning colour over the bandage and cut! We were on stage within two hours of this happening. At the time, it was extremely stressful, but we got through it and we laugh about it now.

Change Your Body with the World's Fittest Couple

At our last competition in 2006, we filmed a documentary about the whole 84 day training and diet process. Four weeks out of competition, I was taking a self-defence session for 17 year old boys at a Catholic College and I was holding a kick bag for a tall lanky kid while instructing and watching the rest of the class. The student was doing a front kick at full power and missed the kick bag. My knees are not the best anyway, and I just copped a full - blown kick right to the front of my left knee. The feeling I had in my stomach when that occurred was sickening. Four weeks out, and now my knee was the size of a balloon. I was shattered.

After the session, I lay down and iced it straight away, and then the mind monkeys started chatting away: "Well, you have done it now, you won't be able to compete, it is all over. All that hard work is for nothing. Give up, you are finished. This is a serious injury and there is no way you can do the acrobatic routine." Many more negative thoughts crept in, but I just lay there with a single thought of, "What's done is done." What could I do to get back on track?

I refused to get it checked by a doctor because I just didn't want to know how bad it was. There was nothing they could do in that time frame anyway, and I really wanted to compete and finish the documentary because it needed a good ending. At that time, I couldn't do the routine and struggled with some of the moves. On the competition day, it was just 90 seconds, so I sucked it up, put on a smile and just did it. When we returned, I went straight to my doctor to find out that I had cracked my patella and had a floating bone in my knee. A little bit of pain and another World Fitness title – it was all worth it!

Chapter 9 — Overcoming Obstacles

The Obstacle in Our Path

In ancient times, a king had a boulder placed on a roadway. Then he hid himself and watched to see if anyone would remove the huge rock. Some of the king's wealthiest merchants and courtiers came by and simply walked around it. Many loudly blamed the king for not keeping the roads clear, but nobody did anything about getting the big stone out of the way. Then a peasant came along carrying a load of vegetables. On approaching the boulder, the peasant laid down his burden and tried to move the stone to the side of the road. After much pushing and straining, he finally succeeded. As the peasant picked up his load of vegetables, he noticed a purse lying in the road where the boulder had been. The purse contained many gold coins and a note from the king indicating that the gold was for the person who removed the boulder from the roadway. The peasant learned what many others never understand.

Every obstacle presents an opportunity to improve one's condition.

—Author Unknown

DON'T let your thoughts become your obstacles. Are you constantly worried about what you are eating, always dieting, or just trying to lose weight? DON'T let your weight or food control YOU.

The more you think about food the more you will probably eat! Get busy, get a new hobby, a new job, or join a gym, and be proactive about changing your attitude toward food. Many people turn to food in times of emotional stress. If you are constantly emotionally stressed then you are not able to reach your true potential, both mentally and physically.

Emotional baggage may be things like:

- Disliking your job – if you are at work for eight hours a day doing something you don't like, move on and challenge yourself to find a new job
- Relationship problems – maybe you need to like and respect yourself before you can like a partner
- Lack of sleep - can make you irritable and unmotivated, so establish why you are not sleeping
- Not enough time for yourself – for example, working too hard, running after kids, it gets down to time management and making time for you.

Letting go of this emotional baggage will make losing weight much easier. Start today, and deal with your emotions. Remember, YOU are the only one that can make these changes, no one else can.

"You are the only real obstacle in your path to a fulfilling life."

—**Les Brown**

In the second year of competition and six months into my training regime, I was jogging about three times a week. The pain was getting worse, and each time I ran, my knees would get more

Chapter 9 — Overcoming Obstacles

and more swollen. I knew that I had to keep on running to better my cardiovascular fitness and to prepare my legs for acrobatics because if my legs could not put up with jolts from running, they wouldn't cope with flipping and landing.

So, after seeing a specialist, I was booked for a double knee arthroscopy. The doctors wanted to do one knee, then the other, but I insisted on getting both done at the same time. They told me that this was not a good idea because I wouldn't be able to move. I told them that I was used to that and to do them together. They would both heal quicker, and I could get back to training. During this time, I still trained; I just did upper body. It was one of the many little obstacles I encountered along the way.

At our fitness training centre, we hear excuses (obstacles) all the time, such as:

Obstacle: I couldn't go running because it was raining. **Solutions:** Wear wet weather gear or do an indoor circuit.

Obstacle: I had to work. **Solutions:** Get up one hour earlier, train at lunchtime, walk to meetings, ride or walk to work, always take stairs, see exercise as a stress relief, use exercise to make you sleep better and quiet your mind when at work.

Obstacle: My wife or kids were sick. **Solutions:** Ring a family member or neighbour to watch over them, book a doctor's appointment and run around the block while waiting, put a movie on for them to watch while you train indoors using the gymstick and rebounder, train inside while they sleep.

Obstacle: I don't have enough money to join a gym or get a personal trainer. **Solution:** Add up how much you spend on coffees, junk food, alcohol, clothes, and cigarettes in a week. You will be shocked! Yes, you do have enough money. See your fitness as an investment in your health, not an expense. No excuses, just results.

> *Never say I can't afford it, say what do I have to do to afford this*
>
> —**Robert T. Kiyosakis,** Author

To some people, my train accident would be an unconquerable obstacle. Believe it or not, it was one of the best things that ever happened to me. The amount of strength I gained from intensive rehabilitation gave me an awareness of how hard I could push myself. Monica and I are closer than ever. We have an unbreakable bond. Besides, the accident is part of my reality, which means I can't change it, so why not use it as an opportunity for personal and spiritual growth?

Chapter 9 — Overcoming Obstacles

The following butterfly story sums this chapter up perfectly:

The Butterfly Story

A man found a cocoon of a butterfly. One day a small opening appeared in the cocoon and he sat and watched the butterfly for several hours as it struggled to force its body through that little hole. Then it seemed to stop making any progress. It appeared as if it had gotten as far as it could and it couldn't go further.

Then the man decided to help the butterfly, so he took a pair of scissors and snipped off the remaining bit of the cocoon. The butterfly then emerged easily. But it had a swollen body and small, shriveled wings.

The man continued to watch the butterfly because he expected that, at any moment, the wings would enlarge and expand to be able to support the body, which would contract in time.
Neither happened! In fact, the butterfly spent the rest of its life crawling around with a swollen body and shriveled wings. It never was able to fly.

What the man in his kindness and haste did not understand was that the restricting cocoon and the struggle required for the butterfly to get through the tiny opening were nature's way of forcing fluid from the body of the butterfly into its wings so that it would be ready for flight once it achieved its freedom.

Sometimes struggles are exactly what we need in our life. If nature allowed us to go through our life without any obstacles, it would cripple us. We would not be as strong as what we could have been.

And we could never fly...

—**Author Unknown**

SECTION 2
BECOME EDUCATED

Chapter 10
– Eat Yourself to Health

"Let food be thy medicine and medicine be thy food."

—**Hippocrates**

Did you know that the human body is a perfectly created organism designed to heal, repair, and maintain itself? It has billions of cells working together in harmony striving for the highest level of health. Why, then, is there so much disease and illness? It is because these billions of cells are not getting the fuel they were designed to receive in the form of adequate nutrition. The way we eat today has changed dramatically from it's raw form 50 years ago.

It is essential these days to help your body stay in balance by living a healthy and active lifestyle, consisting of good eating habits and daily exercise routines. Obesity has become a worldwide epidemic

Chapter 10 — Eat Yourself to Health

directly affecting the health of millions of people. In addition to body image issues, obesity causes significant health issues. It is the second leading cause of preventable death (after smoking) and is associated with type 2 diabetes, heart disease, and certain types of cancer.

> *"The doctor of the future will give no medicine, but will interest his patients in the care of human frame, and in the cause and prevention of disease."*
>
> —T. A. Edison

Life is a gift. I know; I learned it the hard way. Get the most out of life by putting the right foods into your body and pushing yourself to be at your fittest. Don't let disease steal your life from you. Would you rather eat that fried food and wash it down with a beer or soft drink every night, or watch your children and their children grow and mature? Is processed food really worth missing out on your life? We are what we eat! Remember this every time you put something into your mouth. You only have one life to live, so wouldn't you want to do everything possible to live as long as you can?

It's like filling up your car with contaminated petrol. Why put processed food, sugars, high fat foods, drugs, and alcohol into your body and then constantly complain that you are tired, sick, can't get up in the morning, have headaches and feel bloated? Nobody else can do it for you. You are the one that feeds yourself, you are the one that can mentally train yourself and use self control. No one else is to blame!

All the information we have sourced in this section has come from years of research, trials, and testing. It has come from numerous sources all over the world and is now ready for you to consume to become better educated.

In the world today, we watch as humans are becoming fatter and lazier, and it is killing us. We were watching a program on television recently on obesity as a worldwide epidemic. Not just America and Australia anymore, but also in Russia, China, and Germany.

The program mentioned this rapidly spreading "so-called disease" of obesity to be more of a threat to our survival than terrorism! Can we stop obesity ? Absolutely, but we need to do it within ourselves, one person at a time. It involves tackling the problem of addiction, acidity, and lack of discipline.

We were out to dinner recently and casually watched a young couple eat. They had some alcohol for starters, then went outside for cigarettes, came back inside for a fried meal with chips, washed down with beer, went outside for some more cigarettes, then inside for some wine and sugary desserts, then outside for coffee and more cigarettes. So, essentially they had: salt, alcohol, nicotine, sugar, and caffeine. They were not feeding their bodies with good nutrition; they were slaves to their addiction to nicotine, alcohol and processed foods.

Processed fast food is some of the most nutritionally deficient and chemically loaded food on the planet. As Kevin Trudeau states in his book, *Natural Cures They Don't Want You to Know About*, "If the definition of food was fuel for the body that also encourages life, then processed food could no longer be called food. It should be called 'fast

Chapter 10 — Eat Yourself to Health

good tasting poison' which is a more accurate description. If you eat fifteen meals per week in a fast food restaurant, you have a 90% chance of getting cancer, heart disease, diabetes, acid reflux, obesity, and dozens of other diseases."

It is not about eliminating these foods from your diet forever it is about having them in moderation. Remember that good health results from a combination of a healthy alkaline diet, supplements that invigorate your body, and moving the body every day. How you can manage these critical health requirements is provided in the next section.

Even though we are all human, everyone's body and genetic makeup is unique. So, what works for your family and friends might not work for you. Use this book to gather the knowledge you need to transform YOUR body. We don't count calories or weigh our food. There is no need to become obsessive, just become aware of what is going in your mouth. Finally, give our *84 Day Body Challenge* a go. We have outlined many options for eating and training throughout the *Action Manual*, so just select one that suits you and let your body decide what works!

By eating yourself to health, you will add years to your life and life to your years! YOU can and will have the body you always wanted.

> *"Most people get ill for one of three reasons – overeating, eating processed foods or hunger."*
>
> —**Tibetan Quote**

Chapter 11
– Eat Green Stay Lean™

"If you don't do what's best for your body, you're the one who comes up on the short end."

—Julius Erving

Your health must be your number one priority in your life because without your health, nothing else matters – not your family, your finances, your relationships, your job, nor even your contribution to society. If your health is affected, then it directly affects every other area of your life. Time is wasted from illness, money wasted on operations and doctors, and you lack the energy to engage in activities with friends or family.

Chapter 11 — Eat Green Stay Lean™

It is a fact that the body does not know how to use processed foods. These foods have been altered so much that the body does not recognize them as food. If you give your body whole foods then your body will use them, but give your body processed foods and your body will store them as fat or a toxin. Which would you prefer?

The further you get from food in its natural form, the fewer nutrients it has. An example is an apple, full of vitamins and fibre. Then, look at bottled apple juice that has been processed, sweetened, and preserved. The body thinks it is pure sugar. Look at your diet. How much of it is food in its natural form? How much of it is processed, made by humans and not by nature?

From all the books on this topic that we have read, you would have to eat over five times as much food as your grandparents just to receive the same nutritional value! Therefore, we are all nutritionally deficient in some way and our bodies need good quality supplements and healthy food.

There has never been a time in history when we were aware of so many diseases, disorders, syndromes, or illness as we are today. On a global scale, we have also never invested as much money in health care as we do today. One in three of us is likely to develop heart disease; one in four will be diagnosed with cancer; and one in five suffer obesity.

> *"Natural forces within us are the true healers of disease."*
>
> **—Hippocrates**

So What's the Deal?

Is our health care system to blame? No, because it only deals with symptoms of the disease or illness and not the causes. Germs are not the source of the disease. They are there because our bodies are conducive to their existence.

If our bodies are our homes, then the majority of us are living in dumps and we need to do some major repairs. As a population, we are slowly digging our graves with our teeth!

So How Did this Happen?

We run around stressed out, trying to cram everything into not nearly enough time. We work long hours, live off little to no quality sleep, and constantly fuel our bodies with artificial highs of caffeine, nicotine, sugar, and quick, ready-to-eat, processed foods because we have run out of time to eat nutritious food. When we finally finish our marathon of a day, we arrive home exhausted. We crash in one spot trying to ignore the hunger pains we have masked all day with fake food, and by this time we are parched from the six coffees and no water all day. So, we celebrate the end of a hectic day by over-eating: a massive meal washed down with alcohol to quench the body and settle the nerves. Once relaxed in a mildly sedated coma, we stare at a box till our eyelids get heavy and then go to bed way too late, so we can get up way too early, to beat traffic. We do it all over again the next day. Sound familiar?

It is our attitudes we have developed toward our bodies; if it doesn't kill me right away, I will worry about it later, now I just want to have a good time. We value everything more than the health of our bodies, and it is killing us. For most of the population, our bodies are out of balance and fighting a losing battle to maintain health, vitality, and the ability to fight against disease. So how is this modern lifestyle affecting our health so much?

In one word, the answer is ACID.

What is Acid?

Potential hydrogen, or pH, is the measurement of how acidic or alkaline a solution is. On the pH scale of 0 to 14, seven is neutral, below seven is acidic. Above seven is alkaline. The pH level in our bodies is affected by everything we do, but especially our lifestyle and nutrients. A human's internal environment remains alkaline with a pH of just over 7.0.

Every shift in one pH unit is actually a tenfold increase or decrease in acidity levels. Consequently, the difference in acidity between a pH of 6.5 and 3.5 is not three times more acid but 1,000 times more acid. The higher the pH reading, the more alkaline and oxygen-rich the fluid. The lower the pH reading, the more acidic and oxygen-deprived.

Dr. Otto Wallberg, a Nobel Prize-winning author, discovered that cancer, and all viruses leading to disease and sickness, cannot live in an oxygen rich environment. When your body pH is acidic, there is very little oxygen in your blood and in your tissues. Mental and emotional stress affects every cell in the body. The mind can turn the body's pH to acidic in a matter of minutes.

A great example of the impact that stress has on the body's pH is what happened to one of our clients who went for a blood test. He had taken time off work to do this test and had been sitting in the waiting room for 30 minutes. Another 30 minutes went by, and he started to feel his anger and impatience rise. He spoke to the receptionist who said it wouldn't be too much longer, so he rang work and said he would be late. Another 30 minutes went past and he again went up to the receptionist, raising his voice this time. He then had to cancel the meeting at work and started pacing the room, getting angrier and angrier. Finally, after nearly two hours of waiting, he was called in for his test.

Three days later his doctor called and asked him to come in urgently to discuss the result of the blood test. He booked the next day and was informed by his doctor that he had type 2 diabetes. He was completely shocked! After two specialist appointments, he had to take another blood test a few days after the first one – this time with no waiting. Guess what? The blood test came back normal!

Acidity is not a new concept. In 1933, Dr. William Howard Hay published a ground-breaking book, *A New Health Era*, in which he maintained that all disease is caused by auto-toxication, or self-poisoning, due to acid accumulation in the body. More recently, in his remarkable book *Alkalise or Die*, Dr. Theodore A. Baroody said essentially the same thing: "The countless names of illnesses do not really matter. What does matter is that they all come from the same root cause ... too much tissue acid waste in the body. Too much acidity in the body is like having too little oil in the car. It just grinds to a halt one lazy Sunday afternoon. There you are – stuck. The body does the same thing. It starts creaking to a stop along the byways of life and you find yourself in some kind of discomfort. I watch with great concern as people of all classes and lifestyles suffer from this excess". He attributes no less than 68 major health conditions to a prior existent acidic inner terrain.

Dr. Lynda Frassetto, an acid-alkaline researcher from the University of California, says that our bodies do not handle acid waste the way they did previously. Her research showed the sheer volume of acid waste our bodies must handle has forced them to take drastic warlike action to preserve their strategic reserves, the kidney and liver, our major detoxification organs. In her study of almost 1,000 aging subjects, she found that we are now stockpiling acid in fatty deposits rather than eliminating it via kidney and liver functions. The body has chosen to save the kidney and liver from degradation by excess acid. There is a cost to this, though, and it is called obesity, lowered immunity, lack of energy, and a whole host of acid-related diseases to which we are subject, including the big three: cancer, diabetes, and osteoarthritis.

These acid wastes move around the body via the blood and lymphatic system until our overloaded kidneys decide to dump them in fat. As Dr. Frassetto discovered, we dump toxic wastes in fatty deposits as far away from the organs and heart as possible: on the buttocks, the chest, the thighs and the stomach. Author and research scientist Dr Robert O. Young writes that he "sees sugar as an acid and as the reason we are so fat" He says that the body has to protect itself from the excess sugar we consume, and so it co-opts fat to encase it and protect us from it. "Fat," he says, "is saving our lives."

> *"It is not the germs we need worry about. It is our inner terrain."*

Blood is your river of life. It transports oxygen and nutrients to every cell in the body. Your blood must maintain an alkaline environment of pH 7.36 in order to function properly. This is essential for life. The body is quite good at regulating blood pH, given the variety of things that people do every day to upset this balance.

Emotional stress, anger, frustration, processed foods, and a poor, nutrition-deficient diet cause acid in our system, which creates a breakdown in our biochemistry. The acid attacks the outer membrane and weakens the electrical charge that the membrane carries, affecting the red blood cells. This electrical charge is important because it keeps the blood from sticking together so it can travel everywhere throughout the body via tiny capillaries. Acid coagulates blood. Blood has major problems flowing around fatty acids. This acid travels to the weakest points of the body causing us to feel aches and pains due to lack of oxygen and high acidity in body tissue.

The body combats this by using alkaline reserves first and by depositing the acid into fat stores. The body uses fat to protect arteries and vital organs from the acidity. Only an alkaline body will let go of fat.

Once the body depletes itself of alkaline stores, the pancreas produces bicarbonate to balance the pH and the body draws calcium from the bones. This is one possible reason why people shrink as they age and the muscles go flabby.

Scientists studying live blood using a microscope can see the changes in the blood taking place and correlate it with the progression of the disease process. We use a live blood analysis procedure with a qualified naturopath every six months to check our blood and assess whether it is clumped acidic blood or the cells are moving freely. It is an amazing experience to see your live blood on the computer screen and this is a procedure that we would recommend everyone try. You can tell a lot about what is going on with the body by taking a live blood analysis.

Chapter 11 — Eat Green Stay Lean™

From 2002 to 2004, we were following a typical body building diet of high protein (all meats are acidic) and not many greens or nuts (high alkaline), and whenever we got our live blood analyzed it always showed our red blood cells clumping together. Our urine indicated that our bodies were acidic. It was so hard to lose body fat during this time, not knowing that our bodies were actually holding onto fat as protection from acidity.

Once we started our green whole food supplements in 2005, our bodies became alkaline within days, and we no longer had to train or diet as hard as we did from 2002 to 2004 to maintain our lean weight. We couldn't put on weight if we tried and our bodies remained lean all year round. We were onto something that was easy to follow; we had heaps of energy. We weren't moody and did not have to follow a strict high protein diet. The secret to a great body was revealed.

This transformation in our bodies was amazing and we couldn't believe how much easier it was to prepare for fitness competitions. What was once a monumental struggle between body and mind was now in comparison – effortless. From this point on we began researching everything we could on alkalinity and alkaline supplements.

Unquestionably, green foods and alkaline supplements build the blood and make it strong, a necessity for a lean body all year round. By increasing your pH levels, the body no longer needs to hold onto this fat, and can start releasing it and dealing with the acids contained within. So many of our clients have seen this fat loss happen after they started on alkaline green supplements – barley grass and spirulina. Remember that healthy bodies are not overweight. As you start to alkalise, the body naturally begins to seek its own ideal weight.

We cannot stress enough the importance of being alkaline. You must maintain proper pH to stay healthy and it makes all the difference in the world with your body shape.

The primary determinant of what foods are alkaline and what foods are acidic is the mineral content of the food. Foods rich in alkaline minerals (calcium, magnesium, silicon, iron, sodium, and manganese) create alkalinity in the body. Foods rich in acidic minerals (phosphorus, chlorine, iodine, nitrogen) create acidity in the body.

Green leafy vegetables and green supplements such as barley grass, wheat grass and spirulina are probably the most important group of foods on our planet. They are the best sources of alkaline minerals. They are an excellent source of fibre and all of them have the best source of chlorophyll. Chlorophyll is the substance that makes plants appear green, the greater the amount of chlorophyll the greener the plant. Chlorophyll is an amazing blood builder, cleansing for the body and one of nature's greatest healers.

Think green and you are well on your way to achieving the alkaline-acid balance that your body craves and deserves. Now we are going to discuss what causes you to be acidic and ways you can start living more alkaline!

If your body is acidic, you will not lose FAT.

Chapter 11 — Eat Green Stay Lean™

Acid Build Up in the Body - The Big 10 Causes

1. Poor Diet

    A poor diet is one that includes lifeless, processed, over cooked, low fibre, or fried foods. This type of diet sets the stage for intestinal problems and lacks the fibre or bulk to assist in proper elimination of toxins. Did you know that a glass of soft drink is almost 50,000 times more acidic than water? And 32 glasses of water are needed to balance one glass of soft drink? If you do not eat any green leafy vegetables high in chlorophyll or highly alkaline foods such as fruits, vegetables, spinach, broccoli, and almonds, or if you do not use supplements such as wheat grass, spirulina or barley grass on a daily basis, then you are at risk of being acidic.

2. Stress and Worry

    Stress, whether physical or mental, creates more acid. An ulcer is a perfect example of what can happen in a body suffering from excess acid. Under tension we burn more nutrients in a short period of time, creating a lot more wastes than the body can dispose of. For this reason, stress is known to speed aging. Stress affects every cell and tissue in the human body. Studies conducted on the effects of stress on the human organism and its functions keep showing that the link between the mind, stress, and disease are undeniable. Immune response lowers, and the functions of all major organs are affected negatively. Stress robs the body of important vitamins and minerals, and over time, this can cause severe acid build-up.

3. Over-Consumption of Food

Over-eating puts a great amount of stress on your digestive system. Your body must produce hydrochloric acid, enzymes, bile, and other digestive substances to break down a meal. When we over-eat, the digestive system cannot always meet the demands placed upon it. The stomach bloats as the digestive system goes into turmoil. Foods are not properly broken down and tend to lodge in the lower intestines, and vital nutrients are not absorbed. Many people eat their largest meal at dinner time. However, this should be the lightest meal of the day.

The human body uses sleep to cleanse, repair, rebuild, and restore itself. When a person goes to sleep with a full stomach, the body is not at rest. It is actually busy digesting and processing a large amount of food. This inhibits the vital cleansing, building, detoxification, and restorative processes that normally occur while you are asleep. There is a wise old saying:

"Eat breakfast by yourself, share your lunch, and give dinner to your enemies."

4. Lack of Water

Water is second only to oxygen in order of importance to sustain life. Water cleanses the inside of the body as well as the outside. It is instrumental in flushing out waste and toxins. When your body is not receiving enough water, toxins tend to stagnate, hindering all digestive eliminative processes. When you are dehydrated you will crave acidic foods, especially sugar. This topic is so important that we have dedicated a whole chapter to it – chapter 12.

5. Lack of Exercise

Exercise stimulates the circulatory and lymphatic systems and improves the functioning of the nervous system, glands, lungs, heart, and brain, and helps to build muscle. Blood is pumped throughout the body by the heart, but the lymphatic fluid depends solely on movement of muscles to be circulated. Lack of exercise lowers metabolic efficiency, and without circulatory stimulation your body's natural cleansing systems that eliminate toxins are weakened.

Your body consists of muscles, tendons, and ligaments. It is designed to move frequently. Lack of flexibility and movement allows for negative energy and toxins to accumulate in various parts of your body, allowing toxicity to build up. We recommend doing a yoga class once a week and stretching 10 minutes every day, especially after exercise. Every hour, just move the body and stretch or walk around, especially if you are sitting at a desk. The toilet cubicle is a great place for a full body stretch if you are at a conference or work. Just swing your heel up onto the toilet for a good hamstring stretch!

6. **Smoking**

If you haven't done it already, now is the ideal time to give up smoking. It is a fact that smoking causes cancer, emphysema, and heart disease; that it can shorten your life by 14 years or more; and that the habit can cost a smoker thousands of dollars a year. Smoking is a hard habit to break because tobacco contains nicotine, which is highly addictive. The body and mind quickly become so used to the nicotine in cigarettes that a person needs to have it just to feel normal. Tobacco is full of up to 200 toxic chemical compounds that can impact your thyroid health and overall well-being.

Smoking weakens the immune system and damages the respiratory system, making it harder to breathe and decreasing the amount of oxygen in the body. This creates an acidic internal environment. Smoking also affects the look of your skin because it damages circulation. A smoker's skin can look dull and grey and significantly more aged than a non-smoker.

7. **Alcohol**

Alcohol is toxic to the body as well as dehydrating the body. Therefore, it can be a double-edged sword since dehydration can make you acidic as well. Alcohol also stops protein, carbohydrate, and fat metabolism. Until alcohol is out of your system, you will not burn fat. Alcohol can cause blood sugar levels to drop more rapidly. That can stimulate your appetite and disrupt your ability to tell when you've had enough to eat. This can also create fatigue, and your energy level will suffer.

Because alcohol interferes with the body's absorption of vitamins and minerals, it can lessen the body's ability to burn stored fat. Also, alcohol is detoxified by the liver. In the process of metabolising excess quantities of alcohol, the liver swells and may become filled with fat. All these factors contribute to what is known as a beer belly. Your body burns alcohol calories before it will burn stored fat supplies, so it slows down weight loss.

That said, enjoying a glass of wine with your meal is thought to help with digestion, and wine is full of antioxidants. It is also very enjoyable to have a cold beer with friends over a BBQ. In other words, we are not condemning alcohol, just live by our golden rule for alcohol. Drink in moderation, no more than two or three drinks in a session, and do this no more than twice a week.

8. Prescription and Non-prescription Drugs

Your liver can become sluggish from non-prescription drugs, prescription drugs, and cholesterol-reducing drugs. The liver is the filter and cleanser of blood and it is also the only organ that can pump fat out of the body. If your liver is sluggish then you cannot burn fat properly. In our opinion, non-prescription and prescription drugs can be toxic and are treating the symptoms of your condition, not the cause. The body is quite capable of healing itself if you exercise, take whole food supplements and eat healthy.

"He that takes medicine and neglects diet, wastes the skill of the physician."

—**Chinese Proverb**

9. Lack of Sleep

In our opinion, colds and the flu, anxiety, diabetes, obesity, and even cancer are connected to a lack of sleep. There is increasing scientific evidence that inadequate sleep weakens the body's immune system and interferes with our hormones.

Poor sleep habits may be partly to blame for expanding waistlines. Two or three nights of inadequate sleep can dramatically affect the hormones responsible for hunger and satiety. After a night of five or fewer hours of sleep, levels of the satiety hormone leptin drop and levels of the hunger hormone ghrelin increase. As a result, the body craves high-calorie foods. Most acidic foods are high-calorie and the amount of coffee and sugar that people take in the morning to wake themselves up without water makes them very dehydrated.

According to the ancient Indian Ayurvedic medicine, it is best to go to bed at approximately 10 p.m. and wake at 6 a.m. Hormones that heal and rejuvenate the body are released only between 10 p.m. and 2 a.m. Sleep experts say that every hour you get before midnight is worth two hours after.

10. Constipation

If you're constipated, waste backs up and toxins become trapped in your colon. These ferment and decay and are re-absorbed into the bloodstream, polluting your tissues and cells. If you are having a bowel movement every two days, start changing your diet – more water, more green foods, more fibre - and start eliminating those toxins!

Lack of body movement may be the cause of constipation. Have you ever noticed that when you take a dog for a walk they often experience a bowel movement? When you move your body as nature intended, you increase the elimination process. Since most people sit all day, their elimination cycles are suppressed. You should be having at least one bowel movement per day.

Symptoms of an Acidic Body

Mildly Acidic:

- Low energy
- Digestive problems: constipation diarrhoea, bloating, and gas
- Mild headaches
- Muscle pain
- Itchy skin
- Joint pain
- White-coated tongue
- Bad breath
- Nasal congestion
- Strong smelling urine

Moderate Acidic:

- Fungal infections: candida, athlete's foot, and thrush
- Poor memory and concentration
- Viral infections: cold sores, colds, and flu
- Hay fever, sinusitis, asthma, and bronchitis
- Urinary tract infections

- Premenstrual tension
- Psoriasis and hives
- Migraine headaches
- Insomnia
- Depression
- Bacterial infections: staph, strep
- Hair loss
- Swollen joints
- Gastritis, gastric ulcers, and colitis
- Ear infections

Advanced Acidic:

- Osteoporosis (weakening of bones)
- Autoimmune diseases: multiple sclerosis, lupus, rheumatoid arthritis, cancer
- Corroded arteries, veins, and heart tissue
- Formation of cholesterol plaque
- Decreased cell regeneration
- Gout

"Living a healthy lifestyle will only deprive you of poor health, lethargy, and fat."

—Jill Johnson

Symptoms of an Alkaline Body (the kind we strive for)

- Energy levels being consistent and higher throughout the day
- Deep restful sleep
- A fit, healthy and lean body and healthy weight loss
- Reduced cravings and mood swings
- Proper fat metabolism and healthy insulin protection
- Correct oxygen flow to tissues to flush out toxins
- Smooth blood flow throughout the arteries, veins, and heart tissue
- Slower aging process
- Proper electrolyte activity
- More energy by being able to access energy reserves
- Appropriate cholesterol levels so plaque does not form
- Proper calcium utilization to lessen the probability of osteoporosis and osteoarthritis
- Critical lipid, fatty acid, and hormonal metabolism

It is very difficult to get sick when your body is alkaline due to the fact that germs, bacteria, viruses, fungi, and diseases cannot live in an alkaline environment; they need an acidic environment to flourish. Alkaline tissue holds 20 times more oxygen than acidic tissue. This oxygen-rich environment is critical for maintaining health and increasing longevity.

Acids are formed through stress, negative emotions, and poor nutrition. We need vital alkaline substances, minerals, and trace elements to maintain a natural equilibrium. These alkaline substances such as potassium, calcium, and magnesium are able to neutralize the harmful acids and encourage acid excretion.

We have provided you a full chart of all foods and activities that are acid and alkaline forming on the following pages. We certainly don't advocate just eating ALL alkaline foods every day for the rest of your life. What you want to try and do is eat 70% alkaline foods and 30% acidic foods everyday.

It is always best to mix the two together. All protein flesh foods are acidic, so always combine them with a high-alkaline food, such as spinach, broccoli, avocado, cucumbers, celery, salad, vegetables or almonds. NEVER eat an acidic food alone, ALWAYS combine with an alkaline food source.

If you are eating a meal that does not have any alkaline foods in it, such as in a café or restaurant, then do what we do and just carry a barley grass or spirulina supplement with you in tablet form and have that with the meal! It is a good idea to photocopy the acid-alkaline list and put it up on your refrigerator, or in your bag, so you start to remember what foods fall into each category. *There is an A4 size chart in the 84 Day Body Challenge Action Manual.*

Chapter 11 — Eat Green Stay Lean™

ACID AND ALKALINE LIST

CATEGORY	High Alkaline	Alkaline	Low Alkaline	Low Acid	Acid	High Acid
BEANS VEGETABLES LEGUMES	Asparagus, Onions, Alfalfa, Parsley, Spinach, Broccoli, Celery, Garlic, Barley Grass, Wheat Grass, Kidney Beans, Bok Choy, Sprouts	Cucumber Squash, Green Beans, Green Peas Lettuce, Zucchini, Sweet Potato, Carrots	Fresh Corn, Mushrooms, Cabbage, Peas, Cauliflower, Turnip, Beetroot, Olives, Soybeans, Tofu	Corn, Olives	Potatoes, Pinto Beans, Navy Beans, Lima Beans, Barley	

	High Alkaline	Alkaline	Low Alkaline	Low Acid	Acid	High Acid
FRUIT	Lemons, Watermelon, Limes, Grapefruit, Tomato Mangoes, Papayas, Strawberries, Bananas	Dates, Figs, Melons, Grapes, Papaya, Kiwi, Berries, Apples, Pears, Raisins	Oranges, Cherries, Pineapple, Peaches, Avocados	Plums Cranberries Blueberries	Sour Cherries, Rhubarb, Canned Fruit	Prunes, Processed Fruit Juice with added sugar

139

Change Your Body with the World's Fittest Couple

	High Alkaline	Alkaline	Low Alkaline	Low Acid	Acid	High Acid
GRAINS CEREALS	Lentils	Amaranth, Wild Rice	Oats Brown Rice, Millet	Rye Bread, Spelt, Quinoa, Rice Cakes	White Rice, Corn, Buckwheat	Wheat, White Bread, Pastries, Biscuits, Pasta

	High Alkaline	Alkaline	Low Alkaline	Low Acid	Acid	High Acid
PROTEINS		Tofu Tempeh	Soy Cheese, Soy Milk	Eggs Liver, Oysters, Venison, All Fish	Turkey, Chicken, Lamb	Bacon, Beef, Pork, Shellfish

	High Alkaline	Alkaline	Low Alkaline	Low Acid	Acid	High Acid
DAIRY		Breast Milk	Goats Milk, Goat Cheese, Whey Protein	Yogurt, Buttermilk, Cottage Cheese, Cream	Raw Milk	Cheese, Homogenized Milk, Ice Cream, Custard

	High Alkaline	Alkaline	Low Alkaline	Low Acid	Acid	High Acid
NUTS SEEDS		Almonds, 100% Mixed Nut Spread	Chestnuts, Brazils, Hazelnuts, Coconut, Cashews	Pumpkin, Sesame, Sunflower	Pecans, Pistachios, Tahini	Peanuts, Walnuts

Chapter 11 — Eat Green Stay Lean™

	High Alkaline	Alkaline	Low Alkaline	Low Acid	Acid	High Acid
OILS		Flax Seed, Olive	Coconut Butter	Corn, Sunflower, Sesame	Canola, Margarine	

	High Alkaline	Alkaline	Low Alkaline	Low Acid	Acid	High Acid
BEVERAGES	Herbal Teas, Lemon, Water	Green Tea	Ginger Tea	Tea, Cocoa	Coffee, Wine	Beer, Spirits, Liqueurs, Soft Drinks, Carbonated Drinks

	High Alkaline	Alkaline	Low Alkaline	Low Acid	Acid	High Acid
SWEETENERS CONDIMENTS	Stevia, Bi Carb Soda, Chilli, Cinnamon, Curry, Ginger, Sea Salt, Apple Cider Vinegar	Maple Syrup, Rice Syrup	Raw Honey, Raw Sugar	Processed Honey, Carob	White Sugar, Brown Sugar, Mayonnaise, White Vinegar	Artificial Sweeteners, Chocolate, Corn Syrup

	High Alkaline	High Acid
OTHER	Yoga, Massage, Laughter, Reading, Sleep, Facials, Happy Family Life, Relaxation, Meditation, Exercise, Hiking, Swimming in the Sea, Coral Calcium, Spirulina	Antibiotics, Processed Foods, Pain Killers, All Drugs, Smoking, Lack of Sleep, Worry, Stress, Junk Food, Working Overtime, Dehydration, Pesticides, Preservatives, Additives, Over Exercising, Electromagnetic Radiation (power lines, computers, mobile phones)

Lemons might be seen as being an acidic food due to their taste, however, the end products they produce after digestion and assimilation are very alkaline so, lemons are therefore alkaline forming in the body.

Extremely alkaline forming foods that we want to include more of in our diet with the highest alkaline pH ranking in order of pH levels are:

pH of 9.0	Lemons, Watermelon
pH of 8.5	Cantaloupe, Cayenne Pepper, Limes, Mango, Melons, Parsley, Seaweeds, Asparagus, Pineapple, Green Vegetable Juices such as barley grass, wheat grass.

Extremely acid forming foods that we want to reduce in our diet with the highest acidic pH ranking in order of pH levels are:

pH of 5.0	Artificial Sweeteners
pH of 5.5	Carbonated Soft Drinks, Cigarettes, Drugs, Flour, Lamb, Pastries, Cakes, Pork, Sugar, Beef, Beer, Chocolate, Liquor, Coffee, White Pasta, White Rice

Acid waste accumulation may lead to many degenerative diseases according to author Sang Whang "Reverse Aging". He states that "when we are born, we have the highest alkaline mineral concentration and also the highest body pH. The difference in your body at 20 years of age and at 40 years of age is that you have accumulated more acidic wastes at 40 than you had at 20"

Our goal should be to prevent this acid build up in the body and keep our bodies healthy by following our 17 steps to becoming more alkaline.

17 Steps to Becoming More Alkaline

Step One – Food and Activity Diary
Write down all your food, fluid intake, and daily activities (e.g., work, home, exercise) for seven days. Then look back over your seven days and circle your acidic foods and activities by looking at the acid-alkaline chart. (e.g processed foods, alcohol, stress at work, not sleeping)

Step Two – De Stress
Start de-stressing your life! Try a yoga or meditation class, go for a walk in nature, go to bed early, plan a holiday, take a day off, change jobs, curl up on the couch, read a good book, or watch a movie!

Step Three – Drink more Water (preferably filtered)
Aim to drink at least two litres of water per day, or eight cups of water. Dehydration will make you crave acidic foods such as sugar, junk food, and coffee. Buy yourself a 1.5 litre bottle of water and fill it in the morning. Then, make sure you finish it by 1:00 p.m. Refill the bottle and finish it again by the time you go to bed. Drink herbal teas as part of your water intake to help stimulate the liver and kidneys to flush toxins out of your system. Peppermint, green tea, camomile, and ginger are all great options.

An easy way to make your water more alkaline is to fill a glass of water, cut a lemon or lime into quarters, and squeeze a slice into your glass.

Step Four – Get on a Green Alkaline Supplement

Try a high-alkaline supplement such as barley grass or spirulina. Use these supplements if you are finding that you are just not getting enough greens or alkaline foods on a daily basis. It helps alkalise the body and gives us a ready supply of sustainable, steady energy throughout the day, as well as helping to drop body fat. It also contains a large volume of vitamins and minerals! When we get ready for a fitness show or photo shoot we always increase our doses of barley grass and spirulina. It works! Refer to chapter 13 for more information on these two supplements.

Step Five – Choose to Move

In our opinion, exercising every day followed by a rest period helps get rid of waste products and acid build-up, especially if you are drinking an alkaline water such as PiMag. In our opinion, exercise helps eliminate acid by elevating the internal body temperature , which expands clogged up capillary vessels, sucking out acid accumulated deep within your body. This high-temperature blood dissolves old waste products and acid and flushes them out of your body, renewing your energy and health. Exercise also increases fresh blood and oxygen into cells and eliminates toxins through your sweat. Ensure you stretch after exercise to break up lactic acid. If you are just starting to exercise, then walking is great!

Step Six – Have a Hot Bath, Sauna or Massage

In our opinion, hot baths and saunas elevate the internal body temperature, helping to remove acid build up, as mentioned in step 5. Please adhere to safety guidelines regarding sauna usage, drink lots of water, and allow the wastes to be removed when having a bath or sauna. Massage helps increase lymph flow. Increased lymph flow removes harmful substances from the tissues and increases immune function. The lymphatic system plays a crucial role in your body's ability to heal from injury and ward off disease.

Step Seven – Combat the Acid

After a big night of drinking, or being in a smoky environment, or even a stressful day at work – all of which are highly acidic – drink at least 2 large cups of water and take an alkaline supplement such as barley grass, spirulina and a high antioxidant supplement such as super juice before you go to sleep. These supplements are critical to your health and well being and will be covered in greater detail in chapter 13. This will help to bring your body back into an alkaline condition while you sleep. We have not had a bad hangover since we have been doing this!

Step Eight – Wash all Fruit and Vegetables

Wash all fruit and vegetables to remove surface dirt or pesticides. For vegetables that don't have a smooth surface, such as broccoli and cauliflower, chop them into small pieces before you wash them to expose as many surfaces as possible. If fruit has a waxy coating, then peel it off. Pesticides can be sealed in the wax. Cook meat thoroughly to destroy all traces of antibiotics to minimise the risk of food poisoning.

Step Nine – Start Juicing

Buy a good juice machine and make fresh fruit and veggie juice using organic fruits and veggies. Drinking freshly squeezed juice gives your body a huge amount of living enzymes, as well as vitamins and minerals in the natural state nature intended. You will have noticed from the acid-alkaline chart that nearly all fruits and vegies are alkaline, so definitely include these everyday in the form of salads, vegies, or juices. Our favourite juice is a combination of carrot, celery, ginger, beetroot, and apple.

Step Ten – Use Magnets

Sleep on a magnetic sleep system and wear magnetic inner soles. The Earth at one time had a magnetic level (called gauss) of 4.0. Today Earth's gauss is .04. Magnetism is essential for life to exist. When the earth's magnetism is low, degeneration of cells develops. If you are surrounded by office buildings, computers, electronic appliances, high tension power lines, fluorescent lighting, and mobile phones on a daily basis then you are reducing the strength of the magnetic field around you. We would strongly recommend you wear magnetic inner soles or sleep on a magnetic sleep system to bring balance back into your life. You spend a third of your life sleeping; but many people sleep on old beds that are too hard or that sink in the middle, and will not invest in a proper sleeping system. The best thing we ever did was to get a king size bed and a Nikken™ magnetic sleep system. It will help to see it as an investment in your life! It is important to get into a deep sleep where healing can occur – if possible between the hours of 9 p.m. and 7 a.m. – for eight straight hours.

In our opinion, and from our personal research, exposing yourself to strong magnetic fields may shift the body's pH toward the alkaline, increases oxygenation of the body's cells, and thus reduces pain. We have slept on a Nikken magnetic sleep system for the last three years and would definitely recommend it over any other mattress. See our website www.fitnesskick.com.au for more information on these products.

> *"Early to bed and early to rise, makes a man healthy, wealthy, and wise."*
>
> **—Benjamin Franklin**

Step Eleven – Turn off Power Points when not in use

Turn off all power points that surround the bedroom and behind bedroom walls before you go to bed (except your alarm clock!) as this produces electromagnetic radiation and increases toxins while you sleep. This is especially important for children and babies when they are sleeping because they are in the most important growth phase of their lives.

Step Twelve – Check your pH level

One of the most powerful and simplest ways to test your health on an ongoing basis is to check your body's pH. Do your pH testing on a regular basis with pH test strips. When your body has the mineral reserves that it should, the abundance of minerals will show up in a saliva ph test as a pH reading of between 6.50 to 7.50. A low saliva pH reading below 6.4 indicates that the mineral reserves in your body are low, and are being used to buffer acids elsewhere in the body.

If it is out of the proper range, then you can look at various things you are doing or not doing, allowing yourself to make the adjustments in your life that will correct the out of balance pH. We check our saliva once every two weeks first thing in the morning before eating. See our website www.fitnesskick.com.au, for more information on pH testing.

Step Thirteen – Reduce Drugs

Please do not stop any prescription drugs without your doctor's permission. If you must stay on them, perhaps see a qualified naturopath for a healthy alternative or to counter balance the acidic effects of the drugs. Be sure to take an alkaline supplement to balance your body. As long as you are taking drugs, you are just feeding your body acid.

Step Fourteen – Reduce Alcohol & Smoking

Reduce your alcohol intake to once or twice a week and no more than three drinks in one session. Do NOT binge drink. If you are a smoker and haven't been able to give up tobacco yet, then we can recommend hypnosis. Many of our clients have had success with hypnotherapy.

Step Fifteen – Take Marine Grade Coral Calcium

This tasteless, odourless powder may be added to any food or drink for adults or children. Minerals play an important role in regulating the acid-alkaline levels of the body, and calcium especially improves this vital balance. Having the proper levels of calcium helps your body absorb more oxygen, which helps build your immune system. Marine grade coral calcium from Okinawa, Japan, is considered to be the best coral calcium available and contains the highest levels of active nutrients. This is also a great calcium supplement to be on if you don't eat much dairy or drink milk. Refer to Chapter 13 for more information on this amazing mineral supplement.

Step Sixteen - Laugh

Everyone has heard the saying "laughter is the best medicine." This statement is true because laughing is extremely alkalising for the body. When we laugh, our endocrine system releases endorphins and encephalins in the brain. The production of these substances helps reduce the feelings of stress and can relax the entire body, leaving a sense of euphoria.

Step Seventeen – Eat Green Stay Lean

Follow our Eat Green Stay Lean™ Diet in the *84 Day Body Challenge Action Manual*.

All 17 of these suggestions are designed to ultimately turn your body's pH from acidic, where disease and illness can develop, to the healthy state of alkaline. If your body's pH is alkaline, it is much less likely to contract illness or disease. The elimination of excess acid is an important health factor and has been largely overlooked in today's society. If you take small steps to change your body's pH level, you will gain more energy, increase mental clarity, improve digestion, and stabilize your weight, naturally. Your health is in your hands.

"Nothing in life is to be feared. It is only to be understood"

—Marie Curie

Change Your Body with the World's Fittest Couple

The story below is a great example of the importance of de-stressing our lives, meeting with friends, and having a laugh, which as we have learned, is a great way to alkalise your body!

"A professor stood before his philosophy class and had some items in front of him. When the class began, wordlessly, he picked up a very large and empty mayonnaise jar and proceeded to fill it with golf balls. He then asked the students if the jar was full. They agreed that it was. The professor then picked up a box of pebbles and poured them into the jar. He shook the jar lightly. The pebbles rolled into the open areas between the golf balls. He then asked the students again if the jar was full. They agreed it was.

The professor next picked up a box of sand and poured it into the jar. Of course, the sand filled up everything else. He asked once more if the jar was full. The students responded with a unanimous, 'yes.' The professor then produced a cup of coffee from under the table and poured the entire contents into the jar, effectively filling the empty space between the sand. The students laughed.

'Now,' said the professor, as the laughter subsided, 'I want you to recognize that this jar represents your life. The golf balls are the important things; your family, your children, your health, your friends, and your favourite passions; things that if everything else was lost and only they remained, your life would still be full. The pebbles are the other things that matter like your job, your house, and your car. The sand is everything else; the small stuff.'

Chapter 11 — Eat Green Stay Lean™

'If you put the sand into the jar first,' he continued, 'there is no room for the pebbles or the golf balls. The same goes for life. If you spend all your time and energy on the small stuff, you will never have room for the things that are important to you.'

'Pay attention to the things that are critical to your happiness. Play with your children. Take time to get medical checkups. Take your partner out to dinner. Play another 18. There will always be time to clean the house and fix the disposal. Take care of the golf balls first; the things that really matter. Set your priorities. The rest is just sand.'

One of the students raised her hand and inquired what the coffee represented. The professor smiled. 'I'm glad you asked. It just goes to show you that no matter how full your life may seem, there's always room for a cup of coffee with a friend."

—Author Unknown

Now that you understand acid-alkaline a little better, here are some interesting theories from great authors on Acid Alkaline that they believe link acidity to cancer and morning sickness.

Author - Herman Aihara

In his book entitled *Acid and Alkaline,* he states, "If the condition of our extra cellular fluids, especially the blood, becomes acidic, our physical condition will first manifest tiredness, proneness to catching colds, etc. When these fluids become more acidic, our condition then manifests pains and suffering such as headaches, chest pains, stomach aches, etc."

According to Aihara, healthy cells are alkaline, and malignant cells are acidic. Therefore following an alkaline diet, de-stressing our lives, and drinking alkaline water, we can always be sure of giving any acidic malignant cells a good dose of alkalinity, thus preventing many diseases from manifesting! Prevention is the key.

Author - Keiichi Morishita

In his book *Hidden Truth of Cancer,* Morishita states "that if the blood develops a more acidic condition, then our body inevitably deposits these excess acidic substances in some area of the body so that the blood will be able to maintain an alkaline condition. As this tendency continues, some areas increase in acidity and some cells die, then these dead cells turn into acids. However, some other cells may adapt in that environment. In other words, instead of dying, as normal cells do in an acid environment, some cells survive by becoming abnormal cells. These abnormal cells are called malignant cells. Malignant cells do not correspond with brain function, or with our own DNA memory code. Therefore, malignant cells grow indefinitely and without order. This is cancer."

Chapter 11 — Eat Green Stay Lean™

Author - Sang Whang

According to author Sang Whang in his book *Reverse Aging* "when a woman is pregnant the fetus takes priority in getting all the necessary alkaline minerals the mother can provide, since a baby is born with the highest alkalinity. This means that while the mother is sleeping she loses a lot of alkaline minerals, and her blood becomes acidic rather suddenly. According to Japanese doctors, this phenomenon is known as morning sicknesss". It makes sense. Drinking alkaline water and using the highest quality whole food supplements are of utmost importance to keep both mother and baby healthy.

Decide today to be Alkaline:

We have had amazing weight loss results with clients when they changed their lifestyles and used our Eat Green Stay Lean™ diet and alkaline supplements. They finally feel energetic and balanced in their work, home, and social lives. It is the answer, or you might say secret, they have been looking for and a true lifestyle change.

Do you want to know the secret to abundant energy and vibrant health? Regardless of how much you work out and try to eat right, if you can't balance the acids in your body then you'll never feel as good as you'd like. Remember, it takes discipline to have the body you always wanted, but following our steps to being alkaline is like the magic key to help you stay lean and healthy for the rest of your life.

Many clients have found that detoxification starts to occur when they reach proper pH. Bowel movements normalize after years of malfunction, and energy returns. They also experience symptoms of detoxification including headaches, tiredness, body aches, pimples, and other effects as the toxic, acidic minerals are washed out of the body. This is all normal and will stop within a few days.

The most important thing you can do in your life today is PREVENT disease and sickness. Most people wait until they have the symptoms before seeking medical attention. People live their lives with aches and pains and use drugs to suppress the symptoms.

Once you start your most important task, discipline yourself to persevere without diversion or distraction until it is 100% complete. See it as a test to determine whether you are the kind of person who can make a decision to complete something and then carry it out. Once you begin, refuse to stop until the job is finished.

Chapter 12

– Importance of Water

"He who has health has hope, and he who has hope has everything."

—Arabian Proverb

Did you know that drinking more water can help you lose weight? When we are dehydrated, our brains will often mistake the feeling of thirst for the feeling of hunger. This often results in raiding the refrigerator and consuming extra calories.

Dehydration leads to lethargy, premature tiredness, food cravings, and ultimately disease. Every person needs water. In fact, each person needs to strive towards drinking at least 2 litres of water (8 cups) every day.

Are you drinking eight glasses of water each day? If you don't, then you may be at risk of having a build up of toxins and disease bacteria in your body. Through the kidneys, lungs, and sweat glands, water eliminates toxins, loosens waste matter, and dissolves poisons in the blood. So without water these things are staying inside your body, making you feel tired, sluggish, and sick.

Water is the number one thing to fix first in your diet. Many health problems we encounter are directly related to being dehydrated. Monica's sister, Janette, is a doctor who has worked in the emergency departments of hospitals all over the world. The first thing they do for any patient who comes in complaining of pain is put them on an IV drip. This hydrates the whole body in a short period of time. Once the body is hydrated, most of the symptoms are reduced or eliminated. Doctors need you to be hydrated so that your chances of recovery are enhanced. Once the drip is finished, most of these patients are told to go home and start drinking more water!

Coffee contains caffeine, which is very dehydrating. Limit your coffee intake to no more than two cups a day. Each cup of coffee needs two cups of water for the body to hydrate itself again.

It is important to get 25% of your daily water requirements into you as soon as you get out of bed. After 8 hours sleep and sometimes sweating through the night, we can wake up very dehydrated. Keep a bottle of water by your bed. As soon as your alarm goes off, have a drink from the bottle to start the day.

If you are not a water drinker, start with 500 ml (two cups) per day and progressively build that up over four to six weeks to two to three litres to allow your body time to get use to the elevated water intake. Often, during these first few weeks, you may be tempted to stop

Chapter 12 — The Importance of Water

drinking because you feel like the water is just going through you and you get sick of going to the toilet. You have to hang in there because it will balance out. In our own experience with clients, we have had clients lose up to three kilograms in the first week by increasing their water intake. You will feel more energetic, you will notice a reduction in appetite, and you may even notice clearer skin.

Monica is always placing a one and a half litre water bottle in front of me, and I will drink it as a normal reflex. It will be gone in a matter of 20 minutes without consciously thinking about it. By the same token, if it is not in front of me then I will go the whole day without drinking because I'm constantly on the go. So now I have three water bottles – one in the car, one at work, and one in my bag. I fill them up in the morning and drink them all by the time I go to bed.

We had another client who wrote out her diet over a few days. Her water intake said two mouthfuls on one day, and then on another day, her water intake said four cups of coffee, two teas, and six mouthfuls of water! When we questioned her about why she didn't drink any water, she said she didn't like the taste and was never thirsty. Her diet also had huge amounts of sugar and salt, and she always craved junk food. When you are dehydrated, your body will have huge cravings for salt or sugary food. An easy way to stop these cravings is to drink more water. Do not wait for yourself to be thirsty because that is a huge sign of dehydration; keep drinking every 30 to 60 minutes.

Our bodies are made up of approximately 70% water. Water is vital for the growth and maintenance of our bodies. Without water, we can only survive a matter of days. If you are feeling tired or have a headache, don't reach for a chocolate bar or a coffee. These are signs that you are already dehydrated.

If you don't like water because it's tasteless, then a slice of lemon, lime, or orange will give it a refreshing flavour without the sugar of cordials. Water also comes in the form of herbal tea, fruit, and vegetables. Herbal tea is excellent and comes in a variety of flavours:

- Green tea – great alternative to coffee, keeps you alert
- Dandelion tea – great alternative to coffee, can assist in detoxifying the liver
- Peppermint – digestive and stimulating
- Ginseng – stimulates brain and balances body
- Camomile – relaxing, digestive, settles stomach
- Ginger – digestive, stimulating, cleansing

A lemon drink in the morning can help flush out toxins in your body, and it stimulates the digestive juices. Make sure you use a fresh lemon in a large glass of warm/hot water.

Follow this with two cups of water before eating your breakfast – it can all be done while you get ready for work!

Blood circulates inside your body each day, depositing water in the sweat glands, kidneys, and lungs. It collects new water supplies from the bowel. Few of us realise that the body stores water in the bowel. Decreased water in the bowel drops the water volume in the blood, which makes the blood thicker and reduces the effectiveness of circulation.

Chapter 12 — The Importance of Water

When your circulation is slow, the brain doesn't get all the nutrients or oxygen it requires as quickly as it needs them, so a few things happen:

1. You may begin to yawn in an attempt to get more oxygen
2. You may start to crave sweet foods in an attempt to increase blood sugars
3. Sleepiness may overtake you as your brain struggles to satisfy its own oxygen demands
4. If water intake is low, and there is none in the bowel, the contents of the bowel become very dry and compacted, resulting in constipation

Below are the main reasons why people don't drink enough water and some solutions:

Reason	Solution
I wasn't thirsty	Keep sipping on water regularly throughout the day. The next time you go shopping buy a suitable, durable, and refillable bottle of water. All water bottles have a rating regarding the quality and hardness of the plastic. You want your refillable bottle to have a rating of at least five. This number will be located in a triangle on the bottom or neck of your bottle. Lower numbers and any plastic bottles should not be refilled because they can leach toxins into the water and can be directly affected by the sun. Fill it up in the morning with fresh filtered water and take it with you everywhere you go or sit it on your desk. Your goal is to drink it all before you have dinner. Keep taking small sips every 20 to 30 minutes, and before you know it, you will be drinking two of these bottles without even trying! Keep a bottle of water by your bed. As soon as your alarm goes off, have a drink from the bottle to start the day.

I don't like the taste of water	Switch from tap water to filtered water (Nikken Pi Mag is a great system). Add a slice of lemon, lime, or orange to your water. Drink iced water
I don't have enough time/I am too busy at work	Herbal teas at work can be part of your two litres of water every day and a great chance to have a break from work Peppermint is a great hot tea to have after meals since it freshens the breath and helps with digestion. Green tea is a great pick-me-up.
I keep having to go to the toilet	If you are just starting to drink a lot of water, try not to go from having one to two glasses to having two litres straight away. Start slowly and build up. There is no solution to frequent toilet stops. Look at these toilet stops as exercise stops – it makes you get up from your desk or couch or get out of your car! You are being more active and giving your body the best medicine it needs... water! You'll get use to it.

If the above information hasn't convinced you that WATER IS PARAMOUNT, then here are some other reasons why your body needs water every day:

- Water is the main lubricant for the joint spaces which prevents arthritis and back pain.
- Water is a great laxative which prevents constipation.
- Water is the main source of life energy for the body.
- Water generates magnetic and electrical energy inside each cell of the body. Water gives the power to live.

Chapter 12 — The Importance of Water

- Water prevents DNA damage. Water makes its repair mechanisms more efficient – less abnormal DNA is made.
- Water increases red blood cell efficiency.
- Water cleanses toxic waste from various parts of the body and routes it to the liver and kidneys for disposal.
- Water helps prevent heart attacks and strokes.
- Water helps prevent clogging of arteries in both the heart and the brain.
- Water is essential for the body to sweat and sweating is an important cooling process for the body
- Water increases efficiency at work and expands your attention span.
- Water is a good pick-me-up with no side effects.
- Water helps prevent stress, anxiety, and depression.
- Water restores normal sleep patterns.
- Water helps prevent fatigue.
- Water helps prevent aging and makes the skin smooth.
- Water decreases premenstrual pains and hot flushes.
- Drinking water distinguishes between the sensations of thirst and hunger.
- Drinking water constantly over the day can help lose weight without much dieting. Also, you will not eat excessively when you are only thirsty for water.
- Dehydration causes deposits of toxic sediments in the tissue spaces, fat stores, joints, kidneys, liver, brain, and skin. Water will clear these deposits.
- Water reduces the morning sickness of pregnancy.

- Water helps prevent the loss of memory as we age. It may help prevent Alzheimer's disease, multiple sclerosis, Parkinson's disease, and Lou Gehrig's disease.
- Water may help reverse addictive urges, including those for caffeine, alcohol, and some addictive drugs.

If you don't like the taste of water then try a filtered water system. You will never drink tap water again! Most people are drinking one of the following:

- Tap water filled with impurities, such as parasites, heavy metals, and chemicals.
- Bottled spring water, which becomes stagnant and dead after being in a plastic bottle or drum for a period of time. Plastic toxins leach into the water, creating impurities.

Our favourite water filter system is the Nikken PiMag™ Water system, which is both filtered and magnetic water. We have been using this for the last three years and have had amazing improvements in our health. The water is enhanced through a magnetic field when it passes through the tap. This energizes the water and causes it to carry extra oxygen and be absorbed more easily into the body.

www.enikken.com.au/mm

Another great water alkaliser is from Ion Life. www.ionlife.info

About the Nikken PiMag™ Water Filter System

The Nikken PiMag™ Water System is based on the premise that good water involves more than just a lack of impurities. The PiMag™ Water System combines a number of simple, yet highly sophisticated technologies to provide sparkling clear, good-tasting water while retaining beneficial minerals in a magnetic environment.

When safe drinking water is poured into the Nikken PiMag™ Water System, it passes through a ceramic filter to remove foreign materials down to a range of 0.2 to 0.5 microns. The water then moves through a three-stage filter cartridge to reduce chlorine, unpleasant odours, Trihalomethanes (THMs), lead, and other heavy metals.

Mineral and silver-impregnated stones placed on the floor of the storage tank inhibit the growth of bacteria, help maintain a balanced range of beneficial minerals (including calcium and magnesium), and adjust the pH balance to mildly alkaline. The PiMag™ Water System adds a fourth dimension by delivering the water through a high field-strength (1,200 gauss) magnetic tube. To purchase one of these systems visit www.enikken.com.au/mm.

Drinking PiMag™ Water is like drinking from a fresh water flowing stream coming down from the mountains everyday!

Benefits of the Nikken PiMag™ Water Filter:

- Is compatible with the chemical composition of our cells
- Cleanses and energizes the body
- Provides mental clarity due to additional oxygen
- Increases energy and strength
- Removes 99.9% of impurities and chemicals through multi-stage filtration
- Flows through a magnetic pipe that fills the water with earth energy
- Restores water to perfect pH level for healthy bodily functions

If you don't use a water filter, your body becomes one!

Chapter 13
– Supplements Make a Difference

"Until man duplicates a blade of grass, nature can laugh at his so-called scientific knowledge. Remedies from chemicals will never stand in favour compared with the products of nature, the living cell of the plant, the final result of the rays of the sun, the mother of all life."

—T. A. Edison

According to American economist and author Paul Zane Pilzer, we are now in the wellness age. In short, that means that a whole new industry has started because of:

- Shortfalls in our health care system (or sickness industry)
- The dealings of the pharmaceutical industry
- The rise of health epidemics
- The lack of minerals in our soils, and therefore the lack of nutrients in our foods
- Foods laced with herbicides, pesticides, chemical-filled water supplies

These are all issues we have come across from time to time, and the wellness industry has emerged, not due to any single reason, but due to all of the areas that affect our health. Wellness products and services offer many different solutions to these health hazards.

The wellness industry is about looking at these life circumstances and concentrating on what we can do to live a healthy and pain-free life. The whole industry will achieve this through prevention and by looking at the major things that affect our direct health like:

- **The air we breathe**
- **The water we drink**
- **The food we eat**

Chapter 13 — Supplements Make a Difference

Nutrition is, by far, the most important factor in our health and vitality. The specific topics that we will be talking about in this chapter are:

- Essential Nutrients
- Whole Food Supplements

Essential Nutrients

Our bodies require 92 essential nutrients everyday to function at optimal health. Essential nutrients must be ingested through food or supplementation as our bodies cannot manufacture them.

The 92 essential nutrients are made up of 60 minerals, 16 vitamins, 12 amino acids, 3 fatty acids and the most important of all, water. If any of these essential nutrients are absent from our diets for any length of time, then disease and imbalance will result.

Ted Alosio a certified nutritional microscopist and author of *Blood Never Lies*, states "Approximately ten diseases have been attributed to deficiencies of each of the 92 essential nutrients. That's a staggering 900 diseases that are preventable through proper consumption of essential nutrients".

The most important of all these essential nutrients to our health, are the minerals. We cannot survive without them as every living cell requires minerals to function. Doctor D.W. Cavanaugh, M.D. Cornell University stated "the most neglected area yet to be fully researched is the subject of minerals and trace minerals. This is remarkably curious as minerals and trace minerals are the very building blocks of all life forms".

All of the minerals come from the earth and there is no secret that mineral levels have been declining rapidly over the last 100 years. There are a number of factors affecting this from mining, poor farming practices, erosion and so on. The fact of the matter is, our soils are becoming exhausted of these vital elements and is directly affecting our health.

In 1936 Doctor Charles Northern wrote an article that was deemed so important by the United States Government that the U.S. Senate ordered his article to be printed. The article is referred to as US Senate Document 264.

Verbatim Unabridged extracts...

Do you know that most of us today are suffering from certain dangerous diet deficiencies which cannot be remedied until the depleted soils from which our food come are brought into proper mineral balance?

The alarming fact is that foods – fruits and vegetables and grains, now being raised on millions of acres of land that no longer contains enough of certain needed minerals, are starving us no matter how much of them we eat!

This talk about minerals is novel and quite startling. In fact, a realization of the importance of minerals in food is so new that the text books on nutritional dietetics contain very little about it. Nevertheless, it is something that concerns all of us, and the further we delve into it the more startling it becomes.

Chapter 13 — Supplements Make a Difference

You'd think, wouldn't you, that a carrot is a carrot – that one is about as good as another as far as nourishment is concerned? But it isn't; one carrot may look and taste like another and yet be lacking in the particular mineral element which our system requires and which carrots are supposed to contain.

Laboratory tests prove that the fruits, the vegetables, the grains, the eggs, and even the milk and the meats of today are not what they were a few generations ago (which doubtless explains why our forefather thrived on a selection of foods that would starve us!)

No man of today can eat enough fruits and vegetables to supply his stomach with the mineral salts he requires for perfect health, because his stomach isn't big enough to hold them! And we are running to big stomachs.

No longer does a balanced and fully nourishing diet consist merely of so many calories or certain vitamins or a fixed proportion of starches, protein and carbohydrates. We know that our diet must contain in addition something like a score of mineral salts.

It is bad news to learn from our leading authorities that 99% of the American people are deficient in these minerals, and that a marked deficiency in any one of the more important minerals actually results in disease. Any upset of the balance, and considerable lack of one or another element, however microscopic the body requirement may be, and we sicken, suffer, shorten our lives.

We know that vitamins are complex chemical substances which are indispensable to the body. Disorder and disease result from any vitamin deficiency.

It is not commonly realized, however, that vitamins control the body's appropriation of minerals, and in the absence of minerals, they have no function to perform.

Lacking vitamins, the system can make some use of minerals. But lacking minerals, vitamins are useless.

Certainly our physical well-being is more directly dependent upon the minerals we take into our systems than upon calories or vitamins or upon the precise proportions of starch, protein or carbohydrates we consume.

This discovery is one of the latest and most important contributions of science to the problem of human health."

The state of the world's soils were discussed at the World Summit, held in Rio, June 1992. The summit reported the following declines in mineralisation and soil depletion:

- Africa   74%
- Asia   76%
- South America 76%

Chapter 13 — Supplements Make a Difference

- **North America**   85%
- **Europe**   72%
- **Australia**   55%

This decline in mineralization, on a global scale, has led to the poor quality of available fruits and vegetables. In short, if minerals and nutrients are not in the soil, they cannot come through in the plants. Sick soil means sick plants and inevitably sick people. Doctor Lynus Pauling, winner of 2 Noble Prizes, stated "you can trace every sickness, every disease and every ailment to a mineral deficiency".

In reference to Australia, drought conditions further hinder good farming practices such as rotating crops. Due to a dwindling supply, fruits and vegetables are often irradiated, sprayed and processed to enable them to last longer in storage. So to get adequate levels of essential nutrients from today's weakened food supply is unlikely.

The body will heal itself if given the right tools. According to Dr. Darma Singh Khalsa, M.D., author of the book *Food is Medicine,* "It turns out that every major disease has a specific natural food prescription that can reverse its course." About 92% of our population does not get the required amount of nutritional requirements. It's vitally important that our bodies have a source of nutrition so the body can do what it does best.

So how can we get all our essential nutrients? The answer is Whole Food Supplementation.

Whole Food Supplements

According to Alosio, in his book *Wholefoods – The Evolution of Supplementation* "a whole food supplement is comprised of only whole foods. The foods are concentrated and converted into supplement form. Isolated supplements are chemically-produced singular vitamins, minerals, and amino acids. The simple way to remember the difference is this: whole foods contain vitamins and minerals, but vitamins never contain whole foods"

Whole foods are the most natural of all supplements. Whole foods contain all the necessary nutrients for our bodies to function in a healthy and vital state. The nutrients are found in combinations as they are intended by nature, and therefore, perfect for the body to absorb and assimilate. According to Vic Shayne, Ph.D., author of *Whole Food Nutrition* "vitamins never exist in isolation but rather within an interwoven complex of food nutrients and substances along with myriad co-factors and synergists. There are over 100,000 phytonutrients that have been identified in food". Whole food supplements do not separate the phytonutrients from the vitamins and minerals, this allows the body to absorb the nutrients as nature intended. Our bodies actually recognize whole foods and are able to digest them more completely.

There are three whole food supplements that we take everyday. Barley grass, spirulina and a super juice. These supplements have made a huge difference to our lives as we have more energy and are healthier than we have ever been. Whole food supplements are now part of our everyday health plan.

These three supplements are essential to have every day on our *84 Day Body Challenge* outlined in the *Action Manual*. Whenever we travel interstate or overseas, these supplements are always packed to ensure our bodies stay healthy while away, especially in areas where foods may be more processed than normal or when we may be drinking a little more alcohol, like on holidays. This also means we come back from trips away just as lean as when we left!

Benefits of Taking a Whole Food Supplement

- In our experience, whole food supplements reduce weight, blood lipids, cholesterol and contain all the essential vitamins and amino acids that the body needs. This will reduce cravings as the body has received maximum nutrition. This is great news for people who have constant sugar or salt cravings. Feedback from our clients taking barley grass or spirulina confirms that it reduces their cravings, therefore dropping their overall daily calories. What more could you want?
- Reduces acidic conditions such as gout or arthritis: Whole foods contain high amounts of chlorophyll, which is extremely alkalising.
- Balances a diet otherwise high in acidic foods (dairy, meat, processed foods, alcohol).
- Assists in detoxification or cleansing programs.
- Helps digestive disorders such as bloating and constipation
- Balances blood sugar levels
- Improves immunity against colds, flu, viruses, hay fever, and other allergies.
- Improves energy
- Improves skin health in cases of acne, rashes, redness, or general ageing of the skin.

Eat Green Stay Lean™ is our motto for life. Don't let your mind decide, let your body decide – try whole food supplements for a month!

Try our Eat Green Stay Lean™ Diet outlined in the last section. It's a great alkaline wellness program. It is a fast, simple and natural way to achieve and maintain your ideal weight. Excess fat is your body's way of defending against an overly acidic system. If your body is acidic you will NOT lose fat!

You wake up, have a shower, get dressed, have breakfast, jump in the car or train, work all day, have lunch at work, drive or take a train home, go to the gym, watch TV, have dinner, and go to bed. Sound familiar? What part of the day did you actually enjoy the sun or fresh air?

The above happens to thousands of people all over the world. Your body craves the fresh air and sun rays every day. The same craving can happen when you are training more than five times a week with weights or for cardiovascular conditioning. Your body will crave certain supplements to replenish, recharge, and regenerate. But how many people actually use supplements when exercising or dieting? It is impossible to get all the essential training nutrients from food alone.

Unfortunately, not all herbs, vitamins, and medicines will respond in the same way to each person. Be sure to check with a Health Professional. We have personally used each product that we recommend. All our product recommendations are outlined at our website www.fitnesskick.com.au.

Chapter 13 — Supplements Make a Difference

Remember that good health results from a combination of a healthy diet, supplements that invigorate your body and exercise.

A point to remember is that anyone with possible health problems need to seek the advice of a competent doctor with whom this information can be shared. We share this information with you because we believe in it 100% and have seen our client's transform their bodies and change their lives through good health. You may use it as you wish, at your own risk. There are many supplements out there in the market place that do not work and are misleading in their advertising. We have only ever given our bodies the very best and have always aligned ourselves with the best quality supplement companies.

We have listed over the next few pages a number of supplements we personally take every single day, without exception. They have played a pivotal role in our success on the fitness stage, reducing sickness and injury, and maintaining our health and vitality.

Our health has improved tenfold. Because our bodies have improved, our attitudes and temperaments have followed suit. We both still have limitations from past injuries, especially my knees, but I can cope with them now that my body is in better balance, and I know that my body is getting the best nutritional support possible.

Monica and I are now in the best shape of our lives and attribute this completely to the mix of healthy supplements we take, a clean diet, lots of rest, and a daily exercise regime. We have seen similar effects in others who have given this mix of supplements a fair go, and we are glad to present these awesome supplements for you to consider and try because we know how well they work.

Working Out What Supplements You Need to Take:

- Do you eat white bread, sugar, fast-food and processed foods?
- Are you taking prescription or non-prescription drugs?
- Do you drink coffee, alcohol, or soft drinks on a daily basis?
- Do you drink less than one litre of water every day?
- Do you have sugar cravings?
- Are you lacking energy, don't sleep well, or get sick a lot?
- Are you a vegetarian?
- Do you go a day without having a bowel movement?
- Do you smoke?

If you answered yes to any of the above, then the following supplements will make a huge difference to your life.

Whole foods are an investment in your life...
Enjoy!

Chapter 13 — Supplements Make a Difference

Whole Food Supplements

Barley Grass Powder

Barley grass is known as nature's perfect food because it contains a unique combination of all natural vitamins, minerals, and enzymes. The best barley grass to have is one that is organically grown and is unaffected by chemical fertilizers, pesticides, or pollutants. It must be harvested when young and alive, and then dried with cold processing, to preserve the enzymes. Barley grass juice has nutrients and minerals that support life, without the negative attributes of some other foods. The acidic-alkaline balance of barley grass juice is ideal. It has a natural alkalinity that offsets the acid quality of much of the foods we eat.

Spirulina

Spirulina, a spiral shaped, microscopic, fresh water plant, containing one of the richest concentrations of nutrients known in any food, plant, grain, or herb. It has an excellent balance of nutrients including chlorophyll, carotenoids, vitamins, minerals, unique phytonutrients, and all the essential amino acids. Spirulina is low in calories and fat and is a complete protein, containing all essential amino acids, so it is perfect for vegetarians.

Fruit and Herbal Juice

This is a unique organic juice blend of exotic fruits and berries known for their nutritional value and astounding antioxidant levels. No pesticides, herbicides, artificial fertilizers, or genetically modified organisms are used in growing or processing. We call these juices Super Juices and there are a few on the market at the moment. Look for one that is 100% juice, and contains no preservatives, added sugar, or water. A cold process method must be used in preparation. This is critical as the nutrients can be destroyed by heat.

These high antioxidant whole food juices are very important because it is almost impossible for the average person to eat the recommended five servings of vegetables and two servings of fruit per day. You can bet that the average child is not getting this nutrition daily!

Have your whole food mix first thing in the morning OR as one of your six meals. It is a great energy boost. We mix one tablespoon of barley grass powder (protein source) with a glass of water then add 30 to 60 ml of super juice, stir and drink. We recommend that you then wait 10 minutes before eating again.

Please keep the super juice in the refrigerator once it is opened. You can have this mix more than once a day, if needed. It is excellent to have if you are feeling run down or getting a cold because it will quickly help clear all symptoms. We usually take the spirulina tablets mid afternoon for increased energy and for an alkaline boost.

For quality whole food supplements we recommend and use everyday, please refer to **www.fitnesskick.com.au**

Other Amazing Supplements to Include

Marine Grade Coral Calcium

Calcium is an essential mineral your body needs every day. Around the world, there are several cultures that are known for living long, healthy, and productive lives. The Okinawans of Japan, many of whom live to over 95 years of age, drink water which is mineral rich. Their calcium-enriched water comes from coral. There are two grades of coral calcium available. One is marine grade, which comes from the ocean. The other is non-marine grade, which comes from the sand on the beach. Marine grade coral calcium is the most bio-absorbable form of coral calcium and contains the highest level of active nutrients.

It comes as a powder and has no taste, so just mix it with water and it looks like milk. Most calcium supplements come mixed with magnesium.

Calcium and magnesium are two of the most important minerals found in the body. In fact, numerous functions within our bodies are related to these two minerals in one way or another. Although calcium and magnesium can be found in several types of foods, cooking or food processing depletes much of their usefulness. A calcium supplement is very useful for women who do not eat dairy products. The other benefit of having magnesium is that it can help with muscle recovery, if you are sore from a training session. With all the training that Monica and I do, and the fact that we don't eat much dairy, this supplement is vital to our health and vitality.

Coral calcium benefits include:

- Balanced calcium/magnesium ratio
- Improved bone strength and density
- Relief of muscular aches and pains
- Fewer cramps and muscle spasms
- Improved joint mobility in arthritis
- Reduced body acidity for cell health

Siberian Ginseng

The herb Ginseng has been a part of Chinese medicine for over 2000 years. It is used for increased energy, immune support, normalising appetite, and hormone regulation. Ginseng also aids in relieving nervous tension, stress and mild anxiety. Ginseng normalises blood pressure and acts as a detoxifying agent. This is a great alternative for energy when you are feeling low and trying to wean yourself off copious amounts of coffee.

There are 3 types of Ginseng – Panax, American and Siberian. Siberian Ginseng was widely used by the Soviet athletes in the '70s to improve performance and was labelled Siberian Ginseng when it was first sold in the US. We tend to use the Siberian ginseng over the other 2 due to the fact that Siberian helps the body adapt and cope with physical and mental stress.

We found taking ginseng to be very supportive to the demands of our long hours at work, training one-two hours a day and only getting six hours sleep at night. We were also conscious of not having too much caffeine or green tea to lift our energy levels. So a ginseng supplement was a great way to stay energetic for our clients and our training.

Chapter 13 — Supplements Make a Difference

Fish Oil

Fish oil is another important supplement for helping you achieve an amazing body transformation. Fish oil increases utilization of fat stores, decreasing fat storage. A minimum dose of fish oil is three grams per day.

Fish oil has been proven to work wonders for your heart and all the arteries and veins that make up your cardiovascular system. It helps to lower cholesterol, triglycerides, LDLs, and blood pressure, while at the same time, increasing good HDL cholesterol. Scientific studies have shown that pregnant and nursing mothers can have a great impact on the intelligence and happiness of their babies by supplementing with fish oil.

EPA and DHA found in fish oil are essential fatty acids which may be beneficial for healthy brain function, hair, and skin, and have been known to help with pre-menstrual tension cramps and mood swings for females. Split the dosage over the day to avoid stomach bloating. Take fish oil supplements in the morning and again in the late afternoon or at night.

High food sources of these essential fatty acids are: tuna, sardines, trout, cold-water salmon, pumpkin seeds, flaxseed oil, linseeds, nuts, avocados, and olive oil. If you are struggling to get these food sources of essential fatty acids in your diet, a fish oil supplement is essential.

Refer to the chapter 14 - Eating Good Fats to Lose Fat for more information on the benefits of this amazing supplement. You should only take fish oil that is derived from fish caught in the open sea – not farmed fish. Also, make sure the company has tested for mercury and that it contains no more then 0.1 part per million.

Whey Protein Powder

The very first protein source we have is from our mother's breast milk. The single most important nutritional protein in breast milk is whey protein. Mother's milk is 70% whey.

Whey proteins have long been used by athletes following strenuous activity to help the body repair and rebuild muscle tissue. Individuals engaging in regular, strenuous exercise need more protein than those with a less active lifestyle, and whey proteins are often the proteins of choice. It is also essential for anyone wanting to gain muscle or gain weight.

Protein, either in food or whey powder form, should always be a part of several meals throughout the day for the best fat burning results.

Whey protein powders can come in handy as an in-between meal when you are in the car, straight after a workout, or have no time to have a whole food meal. You place a scoop of whey protein powder in a plastic shaker and shake for 30 seconds with water and drink straight away.

If you are looking at losing body fat, get a whey protein that contains less than five grams of carbohydrates. If you are looking at gaining healthy weight, get a whey protein that has more than five grams in carbohydrate. You can also eat a carbohydrate snack with your whey protein powder, such as a piece of fruit or grainy toast.

The two primary times when a fast response through a protein drink is needed are first thing in the morning and immediately after training. In both cases, your body is demanding additional protein to feed hungry muscles. In one case, it's because you haven't eaten for

Chapter 13 — Supplements Make a Difference

awhile, and in the other case, your muscles have been stressed and need help recovering.

Remember that your body can have too much protein in one meal, so there is no need to have a protein shake + chicken or a protein shake + eggs on toast. Have one or the other. If you are making a smoothie, then try not to use all milk, supplement with half water instead.

Use the scoop on the inside of the pack as one serving. You will need to buy yourself a plastic protein shaker, or use a blender at home. Try having a piece of fruit, or a handful of nuts, with your protein shake, to make it a little more filling.

A few ways of having your daily protein shake (you can have up to two shakes per day)

1. Place one scoop in shaker, add two cups water or rice milk. Shake and drink.
2. Mix one scoop with water, yoghurt and ice in a blender – great for a light dinner
3. Mix vanilla whey protein and water in shaker and then pour over your cereal or porridge as a substitute for milk.

L-Glutamine Powder

Glutamine is the most common amino acid found in your muscles – over 61% of skeletal muscle is glutamine. During intense training, glutamine levels are greatly depleted in your body, which decreases levels of strength, stamina, and recovery. Studies have shown that L-Glutamine supplementation can minimize the breakdown of muscle and improve protein metabolism. It can also help during times of injury and plays a major role in the liver to breakdown toxins such as alcohol, drugs, and tobacco. It also increases the body's ability to secrete human growth hormone, which helps metabolise body fat and support new muscle growth

The best times to take glutamine are either first thing in the morning, right after a workout, or right before sleep. A tasteless powder, it can be mixed with water, or added into a protein shake.

Digestive Enzymes

All cells in the body require enzymes to survive and function properly. Taking digestive enzymes causes food that you eat to be broken down much faster than would occur without them; which means less bloating, better elimination, and more energy.

We always keep a bottle of digestive enzymes in our pantry or in Monica's handbag if we are out for a meal. We use them if we eat rich, heavy food or a large amount of food when we are on holidays.

Buy any good vegetarian-based enzyme supplement. Look for one that contains:

- **Papain,** comes from Papaya (for the digestion of protein)
- **Amylase** (for the digestion of starches and carbohydrates).
- **Lipase** (to digest fats)
- **Cellulase** (invaluable in breaking down fibre cellulose into smaller units)

Chapter 13 — Supplements Make a Difference

- Lactase (works in the digestion of dairy products)
- Bromelain (digests protein really well)

Thermogenics

These supplements give you energy to train, stimulate the metabolism, and help burn fat. There are many kinds. Most contain caffeine, guarana, or green tea. Some come in tablet form, liquid form, or you can just have a cup of green tea or espresso. We have found thermogenics to be really useful for a hard training session and for when your energy is low. It is best to take these with a small amount of food such as a banana with 10 almonds, or a piece of toast with mixed nut spread, since some people experience dizziness on an empty stomach.

This supplement is not suitable for everyone, so please consult with a medical professional before taking a thermogenic.

Glucosamine (only needed if you have joint problems)

Glucosamine is a naturally occurring substance in the body with a primary function of stimulating the growth and repair of cartilage tissues after joint injury. Glucosamine is derived from the shells of crabs and shrimp. Most studies show that taking approximately 500 milligrams three times a day for a total of 1500 milligrams is effective in improving joint health.

We both use this supplement on a daily basis – I use it for my injured knees and Monica uses it for an old elbow injury. Also, with the acrobatic fitness routines, we find that our arms, shoulder joints, and back become very sore, so this supplement makes the joints ache less. When we forget to take it for a few days, the pain in our joints returns. We find that taking this supplement with fish oil is a great way to keep joints healthy and pain-free, especially with the high volume of exercise we do. It is also good for anyone with cartilage injury.

When to Take Your Supplements

Supplements	Time of Day
Barley Grass Powder	First thing in the morning or in between meals
Spirulina	Mid afternoon
Super Juices	First thing in the morning or in between meals
Ginseng	Mid afternoon or before training
Fish Oil	With any meal
Whey Protein Powder	After training or as a snack
L-Glutamine	Before bed
Marine Grade Coral Calcium	Before bed or in between meals
Thermogenic	30 minutes before training (not at night)
Glucosamine (for those with joint problems)	With dinner
Digestive Enzymes	With one meal per day

Our supplement product recommendations and where to buy them are detailed on our website **www.fitnesskick.com.au**

Chapter 14

– Eat Good Fats to Lose Fat

We are now going to teach you about the important fats to have in your diet – NOT the ones found in margarine, fried foods, cakes, biscuits, and junk food! Those are all fats that will make you fat. The fats you need to eat every day are the essential fatty acids – a mix of omega 3, 6, and 9, with omega 3 being the most important. But first of all, let us break down all the different types of fat. The good types that our bodies love and the bad types which can be rancid to the body.

Saturated Fats

Most saturated fats are solid at room temperature, and the more solid they are the more saturated fat they contain. They are the most difficult to digest and use as an energy source.

Your body is only able to convert a limited amount of saturated fats per day as energy, the rest will be stored as fat. They are not essential to your health. Try and limit the amount of saturated fat you have to only one meal.

Cut back on the following: grilled and roasted red meats, camembert and brie cheese, deli meats, salami, cabana, margarine, cakes, cream, ice cream, bacon, junk food, and any deep fried meals.

The only exception is coconut oil. We cover this in more detail at the end of this chapter.

Trans Fats

We need to eliminate all trans-fats from our diet. This includes the vegetable oils served in clear plastic, or those that have been heated in processing, or have been exposed to air; all these will be rancid. This rancidity produces trans fatty acids, the most destructive pollutant in the body.

Trans-fatty acids are found in numerous foods – commercially packaged goods, packaged biscuits commercially fried food such as hot chips from some fast food chains, other packaged snacks such as microwave popcorn, vegetable shortening, most junk food and some margarines. Any packaged goods that contain "partially-hydrogenated vegetable oils," "hydrogenated vegetable oils," or "shortening" most likely contain trans-fatty acids and should be avoided.

Mono Unsaturated Fats

Nuts and olive oil are the main source of these fats, and they provide an abundance of protein and essential fatty acids. Nuts are raw foods that contain life-supporting and invigorating enzymes, and they do not increase cholesterol levels of the blood.

Chapter 14 — Eat Good Fats to Lose Fat

The monounsaturated fatty acid most commonly found in our food is oleic acid, the main component of olive oil, as well as the oils from almonds, pecans, cashews, peanuts, and avocados.

Polyunsaturated Fats

These are the most important because they are the only source of all three essential fatty acids – linoleic, linolenic and arachiodonic acid.

Linoleic is the most important out of the three. It cannot be produced by the body and must be supplied in the diet. It has the unique ability to lower the cholesterol levels in the blood and is very important for the prevention of heart disease.

Best choices of polyunsaturated are fish, flaxseed (oil and seeds), linseed (oil and seeds), LSA mix (linseed, sunflower seeds and almonds), walnuts, brazil nuts, sesame seeds, soybeans, tofu and chick peas.

The best fats to eat are the ones that provide essential fatty acids (omega 3,6 and 9), which are the monounsaturated and polyunsaturated varieties from the list above. They have been identified as vital nutrients that our bodies need for various critical functions, such as delivering nutrients to our tissues and other cells, removing toxins, assisting in bowel elimination and supporting skin, nails, hair, brain and organs. They cannot be synthesized by the body and must be supplied by the diet or in supplement form.

As a result, your body actually craves and looks for these essential nutrients in the foods that you eat. If they are not there in the form of flaxseed, nuts, fish, or seeds, then your body detects a nutritional deficiency and you will crave fatty foods and sweets.

Importance of Fish

Fish contains high amounts of omega 3 fat that correctly form brain cells and the lining of your arteries. Fish contains all 22 amino acids, vitamins and minerals such as calcium, magnesium and potassium. It is also an excellent source of lean protein. It's important to eat fish with safe low levels of mercury.

DHA, docosahexaenoic acid, one of the important fish fats, is a constituent of nerve cell membranes. Fish fats have a wide variety of effects on health, including increased intelligence. Fish rich in these important fats are the oily ones such as salmon, tuna, herring, pink trout, sardines, mackerel, pilchard, and anchovies.

Fish oil is vital for the health of the cardiovascular system. Older individuals are less likely to die from a heart attack if they eat at less one serving of fatty fish per week, according to a study presented at the American Heart Association's 41st Annual conference on Cardiovascular Disease Epidemiology and Prevention.

Coconut Oil – A good oil to include every day

Coconut is highly nutritious and rich in fibre, vitamins, and minerals. It possesses healing properties far beyond that of any other oil and is extensively used in traditional medicine among Asian and Pacific populations.

Chapter 14 — Eat Good Fats to Lose Fat

Once mistakenly believed to be unhealthy because of its high saturated fat content, it is now known that the fat in coconut oil is unique and different from almost all other fats and possesses many health-giving properties. What makes coconut oil so different?

The saturated fatty acids in coconut oil are predominately medium chain fatty acids (MCFA). Both the saturated and unsaturated fat found in most junk food, processed food, meats and some vegetable oils, are composed of long chain fatty acids (LCFA). MCFAs are very different from LCFAs. They do not have a negative effect on cholesterol, and they help to protect against heart disease. Medium chain fatty acids also have antimicrobial properties, are absorbed directly for quick energy, and contribute to the health of the immune system.

LCFAs are typically stored in the body as fat, while MCFAs burn up quickly in the body and are used for energy. Coconut oil is nature's richest source of medium chain fatty acids. Medium chain fatty acids have strong antifungal and antimicrobial properties, help regulate blood sugar levels, increases metabolism, and can also be found in human breast milk

Only use organic, unrefined, virgin coconut oil. It must be produced through a low heat process from freshly harvested coconuts. We use one teaspoon each day mixed in with our food. We also use shredded coconut in salads, stir-frys, and porridge. Only use olive oil and coconut oil for cooking purposes. We also use this same coconut oil on our body as a moisturizer!

> *"In the 1940s, farmers attempted to use cheap coconut oil for fattening their animals, but they found that it made them lean and active. If you use coconut oil consistently, one of the most noticeable changes is the ability to go for several hours without eating, and to feel hungry without having symptoms of hypoglycemia (dizziness, moodiness, hunger.)"*
>
> **—Raymond Peat, Ph.D.**

The brain consists of 60% fat and needs specific fats to operate smoothly. A low fat diet, which is almost inevitably low in the omega-3 fats, is linked to depression, and omega-3 deficiency is also linked to schizophrenia and attention deficit hyperactivity disorder. If we add more essential fats to our diet, we can quickly raise a natural antidepressant brain chemical called dopamine by 40 %! That translates to mental and physical alertness, focus, and excitement.

Chapter 14 — Eat Good Fats to Lose Fat

We have outlined all your essential fat choices and the best way to eat them in the table below:

GOOD FAT CHOICES	
LSA mix	Mix of linseeds, sunflower seeds, and almonds – two tablespoons a day with cereal, yoghurt or in smoothies
Flaxseed oil	One to two tablespoons a day, keep in refrigerator, don't cook with it Add to smoothies, salad dressing, or drizzle over vegetables or salad
Fish	Fresh fish – tuna, salmon, trout, or herring Canned tuna, salmon, sardines, anchovy, or mackerel 1000 milligrams fish oil tablets – up to three per day, only if you didn't eat fish
Nuts/seeds	Almonds, walnuts or mixed nuts – 15 nuts is 1 serve, no more than 30 nuts in a day Pumpkin, sunflower seeds Natural 100% peanut butter OR 100% mixed nut butter, one tablespoon per serve – no added oil.
Avocado	No more than a quarter at a time, or half a small one, at one meal
Extra Virgin Olive Oil	Always buy in a dark bottle, use for cooking and salad dressings
Organic Unrefined Coconut Oil	Buy from a health food store, add one teaspoon to all meals or in cereal; use it for cooking Shredded coconut or fresh coconuts are also good, in moderation

The best thing about adding essential fats to your meals is that it creates a feeling of fullness. The essential fats cause the stomach to retain food for a longer period of time compared to low fat foods. The result is that you actually feel fuller and eat fewer calories throughout the day, perfect for changing your body shape!

When preparing for a fitness competition, we are required to get our body fat low through diet and training. We take essential fats right up until the day of competition. It actually makes us leaner and provides energy and alertness. We use avocado, fish oil capsules, coconut oil, olive oil, 100% mixed nut spread, almonds, and LSA mix on a daily basis – all in small amounts and spread over the whole day.

Follow these guidelines to include more essential fats in your diet:

- Use avocado instead of mayonnaise or margarine in sandwiches. Add avocado to salads, spread it on wholegrain toast with a boiled egg on top, and spread on rice cakes with tuna on top.

- Add LSA mix to yoghurt, fruit, smoothies, porridge, muesli, or cereal. Great with chicken. Just cut a chicken breast in half, roll in LSA and herb mix, and bake on an oven tray.

- A 100% mixed nut butter (no added vegetable oil) is a great spread on rice cakes or wholegrain toast. Use one tablespoon for one serving.

- 15 mixed nuts is one serving size. If you are eating too many nuts then decrease portion sizes. Put about 10 to 15 nuts, into a zip lock sandwich bag and take to work.

- Spread your fat intake out over the whole day.

- Flaxseed oil can be taken in tablet form or as cold oil. It cannot be cooked. You can use up to two tablespoons per day of flaxseed oil on salads, veggies, cereal, and in protein shakes.

- Take fish oil tablets.

- Try spreading vegemite on toast with avocado. A great mix!

Chapter 14 — Eat Good Fats to Lose Fat

- Put canned salmon, tuna, or sardines on toast with fresh tomato or mix them into a salad.
- Drizzle flaxseed oil or coconut oil over salads mixed with lemon and mustard.

Other Benefits of Essential Fats:

- Assists in the functions of hormones
- Nourishes skin, hair, and nails via oxygenation and delivery of vitamins A and E
- Increases the rate of fat metabolism in the body
- Reduces blood triglyceride (blood fat) levels
- Reduces high blood pressure
- Regulates heart rhythm
- May assist with reducing symptoms of rheumatoid arthritis
- May assist in the reduction of the symptoms in depression
- Reduces the symptoms of premenstrual syndrome

How Essential Fatty Acids Help in Weight Loss

1. They increase metabolic rate and energy levels, which means that we burn more calories. We should not count essential fatty acids as fat calories because they increase calorie burning.
2. Essential fatty acids help our kidneys dump excess water held in tissues, water that constitutes much of the extra weight in some overweight people.

3. They help decrease cravings which often result from not getting the nutrients we need. Obtaining the missing essential fatty acids satisfies the craving.

4. Essential fatty acids elevate mood and lift depression – a reason why some people overeat. Elevated mood and increased energy also make us feel like being more active.

5. A perfect example of how important fats are in our life is the French diet. It is loaded with all kinds of fats in the form of butter, eggs, nuts, cheese, liver, meats, and rich pâtés. Yet the French have a lower rate of coronary heart disease than many other western countries.

Fats are an essential part of life. Make friends with Fats today!

Chapter 15

– Power Up with Protein

Our bodies need protein to help maintain and build muscles, skin, hair, and internal organs. Protein travels around the body in blood as hormones, red blood cells, and enzymes. The most important thing to remember is that your body can only use small amounts of protein at a time, 30 grams in one meal. The protein that does not get used is simply converted to sugars; then, if not used for energy, it is converted to fat and stored.

Protein has the highest thermic effect of any food. Including a protein with every meal can speed up your metabolic rate as much as 30% because of the energy necessary to digest, process, and absorb it.

Protein is important for the following reasons:

- It is an effective tool for losing weight because it slows digestion and keeps you fuller for longer, just like the essential fats. Always have a protein or essential fat with every meal.

- It helps build and repair lean muscle tissue.
- It can reduce sugar cravings. Many diabetics are on high-protein diets for this very reason.
- It stimulates the release of dopamine, which is a brain transmitter that makes you alert, boosts concentration, and curbs fatigue.
- Protein helps our bodies fight and resist diseases.
- As our hair, skin, and nails grow, we lose protein, hence the importance of having protein everyday.

How Do We Get Protein?

Animal and plant foods are the two major protein sources. Animal protein foods include meat, poultry, fish, eggs and dairy products.

Plant protein sources, although good for certain essential amino acids, do not always offer all essential amino acids in a single given food. For example, legumes lack methionine, while grains lack lysine. What are needed are complementary proteins: various protein food sources that, eaten together, enable a person to meet the standards of a quality protein meal. Always combine plant protein sources to make a complete protein, such as brown rice and beans, grainy bread and nut spread or lentil dahl with beans.

Meats are the most protein-dense food, followed by legumes, and then grains, oats, and rye. If you are a vegetarian, don't worry. There are plenty of options for you without having to eat animal products. If you eat a variety of plant foods – cereals, nuts, seeds, grains, and legumes – you will be fine. You also don't have to eat all these food items at a given meal. You should, however, consume most or all of them during the course of the day to insure a well-balanced protein diet of high biological value. Here are a few suggestions for vegetarian protein sources:

- Legumes such as lentils, three bean mix, adzuki beans, broad beans, soybeans (edamame), and dahl.
- Mix natural yoghurts with LSA mix – linseed, almond, and sunflower seed mix – to increase the protein and provide omega 3 essential fatty acids.
- When making an omelette, use more whites than yolks since the whites have more protein. Give the yolks to your dog – they will give its coat a healthy shine!
- Nuts and seeds are high in protein. Best nuts are almonds and the best seeds are pumpkin seeds or sunflower seeds.
- Vegetarians should supplement with vitamin B_{12}. A 150 milligram supplement should be taken each week. Most sources of this vitamin are animal products, so many vegetarians are deficient. Some vegan whole foods containing this vitamin are: dulse, nori, chlorella, and spirulina.
- Tofu and tempeh can be cut up and mixed into salads and veggie stir frys.

For those of us who aren't vegetarian, we get protein from the meats we eat, such as chicken, fish, and red meat, as well as many dairy products. These foods contain all the essential amino acids we need to help keep our bodies fit and healthy. We also get protein from grains, nuts, beans, and vegetables that provide a limited amount of amino acids. A good way to get the protein you need, and to add a little variety, is to combine the two.

Tuna, salmon, and turkey are the highest flesh foods for protein. Almonds, sunflower seeds, and pumpkin seeds are the highest nuts and seed options for protein. Soybeans, mung bean, broad beans, and lentils are the highest legumes for protein.

In East Asia, the soybean has been used for over two thousand years as a major source of protein. As a snack, the pods are lightly boiled in salted water, and then the seeds are squeezed directly from the pods into the mouth with the fingers. We use this snack sometimes over lunch or as an entrée while dinner is cooking. It is also called edamame and served in Japanese restaurants.

We have outlined all your best protein choices and the best way to eat them in the table below:

AWESOME PROTEIN CHOICES	
Protein Powder	Whey Protein
Soybeans	Also called edamame – just steam them up and eat them
Eggs	Free range only No more than two full eggs per day Use two eggs plus one egg white for omelettes and frittatas
Beans	Four bean mix, or canned chickpeas, or red kidney beans Fresh broad beans, green beans
Red meat	Local butcher is best, make sure it is organic if possible One to two servings of red meat per week (no more than 500 grams per week) Lean mince Lean steak, lamb, or veal schnitzel (not crumbed) Sliced corn beef or ham off bone in sandwiches

Chapter 15 — Power Up with Protein

Chicken	Free Range Chicken breast (no skin); have your butcher butterfly the breast to make it thinner for cooking. Smoked chicken or lean chicken mince (made from chicken breast) Roast chicken (no skin)
Turkey	Turkey breast, roast turkey, turkey steaks – free range if possible
Fish	Canned tuna in spring water or olive oil drained, NOT in canola oil Canned salmon, sardines in spring water, mackerel Fresh fish, prawns, calamari, mussels, oysters
Lentils	Red lentils – just add a half cup to thicken any meal – stir fry, soup, chilli con carne Green lentils – soak first overnight before cooking
Cheese	Low fat cottage cheese or ricotta – half cup per serving Any low fat hard cheese grated – half cup per serving Goat feta – great with salads or sandwiches.
Tofu	Hard tofu is great to add into veggie stir fry Tempeh (fermented tofu) is also great to add to veggie stir fry No more than half a cup per day
Yoghurt	Organic yoghurts only – natural or fruit
Milk	Soy Milk or Cows Milk
Nuts	Almonds, walnuts or mixed nuts – 15 nuts is 1 serve, no more than 30 nuts in a day Pumpkin, sunflower seeds Natural 100% peanut butter OR 100% mixed nut butter, one tablespoon per serve – no added oil.

How Much Protein Do You Need?

The amount of protein you need depends on your age, sex, and weight. We use the size of our clenched fist as a guide for how much protein you need at each main meal, choosing any of the foods from the above list. As previously mentioned, your body can only digest a certain amount of protein in one meal which is approximately 30 grams.

Here are some examples of what constitutes approximately 30 grams of protein:

150 grams meat, poultry, or fish
Two cups of beans, or one cup of edamame soybean
One cup of tofu
One cup of cottage cheese
Five eggs
One scoop of whey protein powder
Three cups of milk or yogurt
90 grams of cheese
One cup of mixed nuts
Two cups cooked Quinoa

Many of our meals are actually 15 grams of one source such as two eggs and then one cup of beans to make up our 30 grams. Sometimes mixing your whey protein shake with milk can increase the protein to 50-60 grams, so you are better to mix with water or rice milk. Try and be aware of eating too much protein and always mix your protein choices to add variety to your diet.

Huge servings of protein (more than 50 grams at one time) is not necessary for muscle growth. If you want to build and develop muscle, follow these guidelines for protein intake:

1. Consume a source of protein with every meal using our protein chart.
2. Eat at frequent intervals approximately three hours apart – five to six small meals a day.
3. Consume a minimum of two grams of protein per kilograms of body weight. If you are an 80 kilogram male, you will be aiming to eat 160 grams of protein everyday, split over six meals. This is approximately 27grams of protein per meal.

When we start to consume too much protein (over two and a half grams per kilogram of body weight per day), we cause excess nitrogen to be excreted as urea in urine. This excess nitrogen has been linked with reduced kidney function in later years. Very high levels of dietary protein have also been correlated with increased urinary calcium excretion. The loss of calcium through urine could potentially be harmful for bone turnover and increased acidity of the body, with the added risk of osteoporosis.

This is even more of a concern as we age and our organs are less efficient and effective. Examples of too much protein would be if you were having more than four protein shakes per day or eating two chicken breasts at one meal. Having a protein shake within an hour of eating a main meal that had chicken, fish, or red meat in it anyway is doubling your protein, and not needed.

The first two years of competition we did it strict and hard – eating way too much protein and little to no carbohydrates. As a result, we were constantly going to the toilet and we would become delirious at times. The final two years of competition, through research and trying different things with our bodies, we became smarter and were able to do it more easily by eating green to stay lean!

In summary, Protein is essential to a lean body all year round. It keeps your metabolism super charged throughout the day, prevents blood sugar lows, helps recovery so you can train more and gives you the building blocks to build new muscle in your workouts.

Whey Protein Supplement

If you are having trouble getting all of your protein through your food intake, then you should consider whey protein supplements. Whey is a high quality protein that comes from milk but is lactose free. Whey protein is derived from the process that changes milk into cheese. It is very convenient as you can have it as a shake or add the powder into smoothies or into cereal. It's great for when you are rushing around in between meetings or don't have time to get lunch. Just take your shaker with you to work with the whey protein powder already in it, add water, shake, and drink. Combine it with a piece of fruit, or a few nuts, for a complete meal!

Listed below are some reasons why you should include whey protein in your diet:

- It repairs and rebuilds muscles after a rigorous workout.
- Whey protein supplies essential amino acids needed for a healthy body.
- It is lactose free, so it is great for people who cannot digest milk.

Chapter 16

– What Carbohydrates to Eat

Carbohydrates come in a wide variety of foods and forms. Virtually anything you eat – bread, milk, potatoes, pasta, vegetables, fruits, biscuits, cakes, and pies – contains carbohydrates. The basic building block of a simple carbohydrate is a sugar molecule, whereas starches and fibre are essentially chains of sugar molecules.

Carbohydrates are grouped into two main categories:

- Simple carbohydrates. These include sugars such as fructose, dextrose, sucrose, glucose – white bread, sugar, processed juices, fruit, and chocolate.
- Complex carbohydrates. These include everything made of three or more linked sugars. Excellent sources of complex carbohydrates are brown rice, sweet potato, porridge, lentils, beans, and wholegrain bread.

Your digestive system handles all carbohydrates by breaking them down into single sugar molecules and converting them into glucose. These are small enough to cross into the bloodstream, because cells are designed to use this as a universal energy source.

There is one exception – fibre. It can't be broken down into sugar molecules and thus passes through the body undigested. This is the carbohydrate we want to include in our diet everyday and has the added benefit of keeping you regular! All vegetables (excluding potatoes), brown rice and legumes such as chick peas, kidney beans, black beans, lentils and pinto beans are the best high fibre complex carbohydrate choices for most people.

With regard to weight loss, you should avoid the following simple carbohydrates as much as possible: white potatoes, refined cereal products, soft drinks, sweets (lollies, candies, chocolate and pastries), processed juices with added sugar, carbonated drinks, white flour, white pasta, white bread, too much fruit, dried fruit and sugar.

How Too Much Carbohydrate Can Make You Fat

Since all carbohydrates are broken down into sugar and are directed to the bloodstream as blood glucose, we have to make sure that we are not eating too much at one meal. When the blood glucose level rises, the pancreas expels insulin to remove glucose from the blood and directs it to the muscles and liver to be stored as glycogen, a useable form of energy. The muscles and liver can only store a limited amount of glycogen, and once those stores are full, the remaining glycogen is stored as fat – something we want to avoid.

Chapter 16 — What Carbohydrates to Eat

Consistently high insulin levels can result in fat storage, water retention, and an insulin imbalance. The consequence of an insulin imbalance is a rapid rise and fall of blood glucose. Your blood is rapidly saturated with glucose, followed by an immediate plummet, resulting in carbohydrate cravings. If you eat more carbohydrates to feed into the craving, then you start the cycle over again. Therefore, insulin can literally make you or break you in your weight loss efforts.

Insulin can be classed as a storage hormone in that it helps to put nutrients and energy sources into cells. Any carbohydrate food stimulates production of insulin. When there is an oversupply of carbohydrates digested, insulin production is over-stimulated. Cells become crammed with energy-giving glycogen and your body stores excess nutrients as body fat.

Keeping your intake of carbohydrates low at each meal reduces the amount of insulin released. Having some insulin release is important for nutrients to reach your cells.

Always remember to have a serving of protein or essential fat with your servings of carbohydrates – the rest of the meal should be vegetables or salad. The added protein and fat will keep your insulin from shooting sky high and keep blood sugars stable. Consistent levels of increased insulin from eating too much carbohydrate in one go are linked with binges due to the carbohydrate cravings it causes.

A serving of carbohydrates at breakfast or lunch should be no bigger than one cup or two pieces of grainy bread. Fill the rest of your meal up with more vegetables, a salad, and a source of protein such as fish, chicken, lean beef, or beans.

We have outlined all the best carbohydrate choices to have before 6:00 p.m. every day, as well as the ones you want to avoid at all times, if possible, in the table below:

CARBOHYDRATES THAT ARE ALLOWED (<u>AVOID</u> AFTER 6 P.M.)	CARBOHYDRATES TO AVOID AT ALL TIMES
All fresh whole fruit – no more than two per day	Bottled fruit juice with added sugar
All frozen whole fruit with no additives	Canned or dried fruit
All fresh and frozen vegetables	White flours of any kind
Rice cakes, mountain bread, wholemeal pita	Potato flour
All beans and lentils, not baked beans	White pasta
Oats, millet, couscous, quinoa, spelt	White breads, focaccia
Whole grainy breads, rye sourdough	Most pizza bases – use wholemeal pita
Chick pea or split pea flours	Sugar in all forms
White rice – Japanese nori rolls only	Muesli bars
Brown or wild rice – one cup cooked only	Chocolate
Muesli bars which include nuts and no dried fruit	Soft drinks, including diet drinks
Rice noodles	Most packet foods
High fibre cereals (four grams of fibre per serving)	Junk food

Our opinion on alcohol intake has always been in *moderation*. Reduce your alcohol intake to no more than two to three glasses per session and no more than twice per week. If you are having alcohol, even in moderation, then remember it is essential that you balance your body with an alkaline supplement such as spirulina, wheat grass, barley grass or a super juice. One of the most important things to remember with drinking alcohol is that alcohol itself doesn't end up as fat. The body burns the by product of alcohol as fuel first instead of burning your fat stores for energy. The result is a build up of fat – not something we are trying to achieve.

Overeating puts a great amount of stress on your digestive system. It is a lot easier to overeat when you just eat carbohydrates than it is when you are served up chicken salad or beef stir fry. Your body must produce hydrochloric acid, enzymes, bile, and other digestive factors to break down a meal. When we overeat, the digestive system cannot always meet the demands placed upon it. The stomach bloats as the digestive system goes into turmoil. Foods are not properly broken down and tend to lodge in the lower intestines, and vital nutrients are not absorbed. When we eat a lot of carbohydrates such as pasta, pizza, or noodle-based meals, they tend to be massive meals with little protein, or veggies, or salad. By reducing our carbohydrate intake and increasing our servings of vegetable and salad, we dramatically reduce our overeating.

White rice, for example, is converted almost immediately to blood sugar, causing energy levels to spike and decrease rapidly, as well as weight gain. Brown rice, on the other hand, is digested more slowly, causing a more subtle change in blood sugar. Processing carbohydrates removes the fibre, vitamins, and minerals, leaving mostly starch.

Sugar is added to most processed foods. Avoid these at all costs. When combined, sugar and flour become even more addictive, such as in biscuits, pastries, white bread, sugary cereals and cakes. Add in all the harmful additives that get put into processed foods and you have a recipe for disaster! In our opinion, they are more like drugs than foods.

According to author Ted Alosio in *Blood Never Lies* "in 1900 the consumption of sugar in North America was approximately half a pound per person per year. In 2004 it was half a pound of sugar per person per *day!* This is staggering and a classic example that we are eating far too many processed foods"

We don't need sugar to survive. But if you need to satisfy a sweet tooth, you can do it without ruining a diet or ingesting artificial ingredients by eating fresh fruit with a handful of nuts! It will provide you with fibre, fill you up, keep you regular, and provide essential vitamins, and minerals.

Carbohydrates from white bread, pastries, cakes, biscuits and other highly processed foods may contribute to weight gain and interfere with weight loss, but that doesn't mean all carbohydrates are suspect. They are an important part of a healthy diet – but only if you eat the right ones. Carbohydrates give your body the fuel it needs for physical activity and for proper organ function. The best sources of carbohydrates – fruits, vegetables, and whole grains – give you essential vitamins and minerals, fibre, and a ton of important phytonutrients. Whenever possible, replace highly processed grains, cereals, and sugars with minimally processed whole-grain products.

Carbohydrates Do's and Don'ts

Carbohydrates on their own digest really quickly and also create a huge release of insulin. A side-effect of insulin, however, is an increase in appetite. That causes most people to eat again not long after eating a high-carbohydrate meal. This means you end up eating more food as you are always hungry, not a good situation if you want to lose weight.

Chapter 16 — What Carbohydrates to Eat

So what is the answer to reducing our insulin and overeating throughout the day?

NEVER EAT CARBOHYDRATES ON THEIR OWN, ALWAYS COMBINE CARBOHYDRATES WITH A PROTEIN OR ESSENTIAL FAT.

This is the number one rule to follow in our Eat Green Stay Lean™ diet, and if adhered to will get you fast results. You will never go hungry again!

Have you ever had just a piece of toast, a high carbohydrate cereal or a muffin for breakfast and then been hungry within 30 minutes? Many people are in this trap and go looking for the biscuits or another muffin at morning tea time. This is easy to fix.

Understand that once the hunger response hits our brains, we literally go into survival mode and will eat anything! The key is to eat regularly and always plan your meals for the day.

Always look at what you are eating and make sure there is an essential fat or protein with the meal. Fats and protein, unlike carbohydrates, have a high satiety factor. Whereas carbohydrates make you hungry a couple of hours after eating, fats and protein make you full and the satiety lasts for hours.

Use our list of protein and essential fats from the last two chapters to help with your choices. For example, if you are used to having toast with jam, then add low fat cottage cheese, eat your toast with nuts, or have a protein shake with your toast. If you are used to having vegemite on toast, then add avocado on top. This rule means you cannot eat fruit on its own, so you must always have fruit with one of the choices from the protein or essential fat list. Fruit is great with nuts, yoghurt, a protein shake, or low fat cheese.

Your dinner should be the lightest meal of the day since we don't need energy from carbohydrates to watch TV and sleep! But for most people, this is their largest meal of the day and very carbohydrate-based. Remember to only use carbohydrate foods for energy –work, exercise, and during the day. Restrict carbohydrates at night, and that includes fruit. Your night-time meal should be a protein source from the protein choices in the last chapter and combined with a large salad or veggie stir fry. Soups are perfect in the winter. We have given you a complete list of breakfast, lunch, and dinner options in the last part of this book in the Stay Dedicated section.

Today, some popular diets treat carbohydrates as if they are the sole cause of all body fat and excess weight gain. This is not the case. Your body needs complex carbohydrates . . . just during the day, not at night!

Chapter 17

– Foods and Habits that Stop You from Losing Weight

"Forget past mistakes. Forget failures. Forget everything except what you're going to do now and do it."

—**William Durant,** founder of General Motors

Our SECRET for dropping weight and keeping it off for the rest of your life is not dieting, excessive exercise and counting calories. That's too hard!

It is eating lots of healthy food that has not been processed, enjoying food & drink in moderation, moving the body everyday and having an alkaline supplement.

In this chapter, we have listed our top 10 foods and habits that we believe *STOP* you from getting in the best shape of your life.

1. NOT Reading Food Labels

Spending an extra 10 minutes in the supermarket, reading the backs of product labels, can be the difference between putting on weight and staying slim and healthy! If you do this every time you shop, then you are learning a little each time about food. Remember, knowledge is power!

When reading labels, look for words ending in "ose" – such as glucose, maltose, and lactose – because these are all forms of sugar. Breakfast cereals contain anything from 0% to 50% sugar. Try to find a breakfast cereal that has no dried fruit (high in natural sugars) and plenty of nuts, these are normally found in the health food aisle. Check the details on the pack before buying. If something is 98% fat free, you can bet it is high in sugar or carbohydrates. Just check the labels first and remember that nutritious nuts are essential fats that our body needs. Eat nuts instead of dried fruit any day.

Other names for sugar on the back of labels are brown sugar, raw sugar, molasses, corn syrup, fruit juice concentrate, glucose, dextrose, fructose, invert sugar, lactose, maltose, sucrose, syrup, and honey.

The order of the ingredients listed on the back of a product state the highest ingredient in the product down to the least found ingredient. For example, in whole-grain mustard, the list of ingredients is: mustard seed 29%, salt, sugar, food acid, herbs, spices, garlic. So, we can assume that whole-grain mustard contains a lot of salt and sugar,

Chapter 17 — Foods and Habits that Stop You from Losing Weight

since they are second and third in the list after 29% mustard seeds. Some hot mustard also contains oil as the second ingredient. If the list of ingredients is long, there's probably a lot of chemical additives in the product.

Did you know that companies pay to have their products placed on the middle of the shelf where you will see them first? The best product is not always the one on special, or the most expensive. Make sure you compare prices and labels for the best choice.

Put your health first. Look for the words 100% organic and read the ingredient list. If there is anything there that you can not pronounce and is not a food, then don't buy it! Do not be deceived by words such as "all natural," "fat free," "light," and "healthy." Read the ingredients list and decide for yourself.

Try to shop at local markets, if possible buy organic, and always buy free range if possible. I have a client named Andy who owns a large organic food business. He literally looks 10 years younger than his true age. He is always lean, vibrant, smiling, and full of energy. Remember, you are what you eat!

"If you still have a slight sensation of hunger after a meal – you have eaten well. If you feel full – you have poisoned yourself."

—Hippocrates.

2. Eating Too Much Salt

If you want a toned body, you need to reduce your salt intake. A safe and adequate sodium intake is approx. 600 to 1,000 milligrams per day. An example of this, so you can understand better, is 600 milligrams = half teaspoon. However, salt is very heavily consumed in the Australian diet, especially in processed foods. Most Australians consume between 4,000 and 6,000 milligrams daily, especially through processed packaged foods and junk food, which are very high in sodium and fat.

Sodium has a lot to do with water balance in the body. Excess intake of salt will cause cells and tissues to retain excess fluid, leading to overweight conditions and causing your body to look puffy – a look that we all want to avoid. It can also aggravate and cause high blood pressure.

The only salt to have with meals and cooking is organic sea salt, which is a rich source of minerals. The mineral composition of organic sea salt is almost identical to that of the human body. When we eat this salt, it does not cause any mineral imbalances and does not cause us to hold fluid. Authentic sea salt should be labelled organic and should be a light grey colour.

We didn't realise until our second year of fitness competitions that salt was affecting our body condition. By eliminating excess salt and high-sodium natural foods from our diet, we started to look much leaner on stage.

Packet instant soups are very high in salt! I know it is easy to do at work, but it is a powder with very few nutrients. Make your own. Just boil up a soup mix full of barley, legumes, celery, tomato paste,

Chapter 17 — Foods and Habits that Stop You from Losing Weight

leeks, cabbage, chicken or beef stock, and carrots for a delicious soup you can eat anytime! Simmer for three hours and process in a blender. Our refrigerator at home always has a big bowl of soup in it. For those times when we are too busy, a little too lazy, or when Monica is away, we always have the soup. It stops me from ordering the Bachelor's Roast (pizza).

3. Be Aware of Food Additives

Monosodium Glutamate (MSG) and Aspartame (artificial sweetener) are 2 food additives you want to avoid if possible. They have been scientifically proven to cause all sorts of physical and medical problems and increase appetite. If you are sensitive to MSG, then look for the additive number 621 on food labels. Many Thai, Chinese, and Malaysian restaurants use MSG in their meals. Just request a meal minus MSG and salt for a healthy alternative.

Try not to use artificial sweeteners. They are synthetic chemicals. Use only organic raw honey or the herb stevia. Stevia is a herbal sweetener made from extracts from the stevia plant. It contains no calories and can be found at all health food stores.

Please note, it's difficult to avoid artificial sweeteners if you are taking a Protein Powder. The artificial sweeteners in Protein Powders enable the product to retain its quality and lifespan. A quality Protein Powder taken as part of a nutritious diet and exercise plan will far outweigh the intake of artificial sweeteners. Please refer to Chapter 13 - Supplements Make a Difference. Taking quality wholefood supplements can actually offset the acidity of taking the artificial sweeteners in Protein Powders.

If you see any of the following additives, sweeteners or preservatives on the back of a food label, try and avoid the product:

- Aspartame 951
- Sucralose 955
- Saccharin 954
- Acesulphame K 950
- Alitame 956
- Sorbitol 420
- Mannitol 421
- Xylitol 965
- Maltitol 967
- Isomalt 953
- Polydextrose 1200
- Thaumatin 957
- High Fructose Corn Syrup
- Hydrogenated or partially Hydrogenated Oils and Fats
- E102 Tartrazine – coloring
- E635 Disodium 5-ribonucleotide – flavouring
- E211 Sodium Benzoate – preservative
- Monosodium Glutamate (MSG)

Chapter 17 — Foods and Habits that Stop You from Losing Weight

4. Cow's Milk

Milk is very different from what it was 50 years ago when cows were milked by humans and the milk was delivered in a glass bottle on the doorstep with cream on top! According to author Kevin Trudeau, cows in nature produce four litres of milk every day. Today's modern dairy cows produce up to 40 litres of milk per day! Cows in nature live 20 to 25 years; cows in dairy production live only 4 - 5 years.

Homogenising was developed to reduce the fat particles to such a fine extent that they no longer separate out, allowing milk to last longer on the shelf. Homogenisation is when the cream or milk fat that normally rises to form a creamy layer is evenly distributed throughout the fluid. This can affect digestion and can clog up the bowel.

Pasteurisation is the process of heating milk and cooling it quickly to destroy harmful micro-organisms that may be present. If you heat food to more than 50 degrees Celsius, the enzymes required for the assimilation of calcium are destroyed. Pasteurisation heats the milk to between 55 to 77 degrees Celsius!

No wonder so many people are lactose intolerant or have trouble digesting milk! It is completely different to what was consumed 50 years ago, and we are still in the mindset that we need milk for calcium. You don't need to drink cow's milk to get your calcium!

Cow's milk that is pasteurised, homogenized, and processed is very hard to digest, even by people with strong digestion. Mother's milk is important for babies, but in our opinion, and from our experience with clients, milk products need to be phased out of our diets altogether.

Try these alternatives to cow's milk:

- Rice milk
- Soy milk
- Goat milk

Great Sources of Calcium other than Milk

- Sardines, tofu, salmon
- Almonds, brazil nuts, sunflower seeds, hazelnuts
- Amaranth grain, sesame seed
- Parsley, watercress, spirulina, barley grass
- Black beans, pinto beans
- Dried seaweeds – nori, kombu, wakame, kelp, hijiki, arame
- Marine Grade Coral Calcium Supplement

Calcium Inhibitors

- Coffee, soft drinks, and diuretics
- Protein excess – especially from meat
- Refined sugars
- Excess concentrated sugar or sweetly flavoured foods
- Alcohol, marijuana, cigarettes, and recreational drugs
- Too little or too much exercise
- Excess salt

Chapter 17 — Foods and Habits that Stop You from Losing Weight

5. Are You Getting Enough Fibre?

The liver is your body's best filter of toxins. Everything from caffeine, alcohol, pesticide residues, heavy metals, and prescription medications are filtered out of your body. If we eat a high fibre diet, we can actually help this filtering process even more. Foods high in fibre fill you up as well so you end up eating less over the whole day, so aim to have every day.

The best choices for fibre are fruits, vegetables, oats, bran, nuts, legumes, flaxseed and beans. Remember that you also need to drink at least two litres of water every day to help this process.

6. Reduce Alcohol Intake

If you are drinking alcohol everyday, this is definitely stopping you from losing weight. Follow these tips to reduce your alcohol intake:

- Make your first drink a large glass of ice water.
- Alternate alcoholic and non-alcoholic drinks at functions.
- Do not stand next to the food or drink table at functions.
- Choose a mocktail (non-alcoholic drink) rather than a cocktail.
- Avoid getting in shot contests.
- Only drink alcohol with meals.
- Choose low-alcohol beers and low calorie spirits such as vodka.
- If you drink to relax or reduce stress, try an alternate activity like going for a walk, exercising, ringing a friend, or reading a good book.
- Don't eat salty snacks with alcohol because they will make you drink more, which explains the peanuts on the bar.

- If you know you are going to have a couple of drinks that day, then make sure you get a training session in to balance the day and help burn the calories.
- After a night of drinking, have a vitamin B and alkaline supplement such as barley grass or spirulina with a large glass of water BEFORE bed.
- Say NO to all pastry or fried finger food – decide this before you leave the house!
- Eat a meal before you go out so that your stomach is not empty.
- Don't keep alcohol at home in the pantry or refrigerator, only buy alcohol on special occasions.
- Enjoy Alcohol in moderation, once or twice a week only, and NO binge drinking.

7. The Salt-Sugar Cycle

Your body is always trying to maintain a balance. So, when you go on a sugar binge, according to Ayurvedic medicine, your body will crave salty foods to balance itself out. We see this all the time in our client's diets. A classic example is after a big night out drinking (sugar), your body always craves the junk fatty foods (salt) to feel balanced. Monica has never been a huge sugar-craving person, and to this day, cannot understand how anyone can eat a whole chocolate bar! However, anytime she has Chinese or Thai food (salty meals), I guarantee that within 30 minutes, she will be craving a bit of chocolate or apple juice (sugar). That is her body trying to balance itself out.

So, if you are constantly getting sugar cravings, especially after dinner, check if your last meal was salty. You don't have to add salt to things for a dinner to be salty. Things like marinades, feta cheese,

Chapter 17 — Foods and Habits that Stop You from Losing Weight

salami, olives, cheese, and take away are all high-salt foods. In some of our clients' food diaries you can almost draw a daily graph of sugar, salt, sugar, salt, sugar, salt… – it is an endless cycle. You can stop the cycle, however, by drinking more water and eliminating processed, high-sodium foods.

8. Portion Sizes

How much you eat in one meal is totally related to how big your stomach is. If you are strict for seven days and eat five to six small meals over the whole day, your stomach will shrink. If you are constantly eating large amounts of food, you are always going to be hungry because you have stretched your stomach! A perfect example of this is Christmas lunch or another big holiday meal. Most people would eat too much food and promise themselves that the next day they will not eat or only eat small meals. The next morning they wake up and are very hungry! Why? After eating such a large meal, the stomach was forced to stretch. The food had been digested and the stomach remains larger than normal. You actually require more food to fill it up than before. This can be a dangerous cycle if you are eating very large meals.

If you only do one thing with your food, do this: Eat small meals, preferably five to six per day! It is the key to losing weight, losing the gut, and having an endless supply of energy all day long.

9. Wheat

We have had many clients, including Monica, go on a wheat-free diet with amazing changes to their bodies. If you have any problems with bloating, holding weight around your stomach, or constipation, then we would definitely recommend that you go on a wheat-free diet. Many people find wheat very hard to digest, hence the problems with constipation and bloating.

Anything with wheat in the ingredients must be eliminated from the diet. That means most regular breads, cereals, pasta, cous cous, cakes, pastries, and biscuits. Instead, enjoy rice, rice cakes, lentils, wheat free breads, oats, rye, barley, buckwheat and quinoa.

This advice is not hard to follow, and once you see the benefits of a flatter stomach you will be hooked for life! It also gives you a good excuse not to eat all the junk processed cakes and fried foods since they all contain wheat – a perfect excuse!

10. Eating Certain Foods Before You Train

Many trainers believe it is better for fat burning to exercise on an empty stomach first thing in the morning. We did that for the first 12 months of competition training and found ourselves to be light-headed and unable to give the session 100% due to a lack of energy. For the last five years, we always have a light breakfast, such as a piece of grainy toast with mixed nut spread, or a super juice and barley grass drink. Add an espresso, green tea, or ginseng and you are all set to go! We got amazing results because we had the energy from that little snack to push harder in our sessions, therefore burning more calories! Now, on the other hand, we do have clients who train better without eating. They have tried both and perform better on an empty stomach. So, this is something you may need to consider. If you are feeling dizzy or nauseous, then eating before training is definitely for you.

Chapter 18
– Mood Foods and Special Occasions

How many times have you woken up and felt great, but after lunch, you felt down and tired? Eating certain foods could improve your mood and provide uplifting energy. First we need to understand the connection between the food we eat, our mood, and our level of alertness. The brain communicates by chemical substances passed from one nerve cell to the next. These chemicals, called neurotransmitters, are made in the brain from the food we eat. The neurotransmitters that are most sensitive to diet and most influential in affecting mood are:

- Dopamine and norepinephrine. These are the alertness chemicals. When they are produced, we think and react more quickly; we feel more motivated, are more attentive, and generally more mentally energetic.
- Serotonin. This is the calming and relaxing chemical. When produced, feelings of stress and tension decrease; we feel sleepy and/or sluggish and our reaction time is slower.

Foods That Make You Feel Alert

To feel alert, you need to eat meals that contain protein, are low in saturated fat, and contain a small amount of complex carbohydrates that won't drag you down. Lunchtime is when your brain's supply of dopamine and norepinephrine is beginning to wear off. When you supply tyrosine from eating protein, your brain will transform the tyrosine into more of the two alertness neurotransmitters, dopamine and norepinephrine. Examples of some protein-packed foods include:

- Fish
- Poultry (without skin)
- Very lean beef (trimmed)
- Low-fat cottage cheese or cheese
- Organic yoghurt
- Eggs

Enjoy any of the above in a grainy bread sandwich, mixed with rice, in a soup, in a big salad, or stir fried with vegetables.

Foods That Make You Feel Calm

Carbohydrates have a calming affect. This depends, though, on which type you eat. Eating complex carbohydrates like brown rice and whole grains will promote the more focused and calming aspect of serotonin release, while eating carbohydrates like sugary snacks, white bread, and pasta will leave you feeling sluggish.

More Good Mood Foods

- Eggs, liver, beef. These foods make you feel smarter because they contain choline.
- Oats. Foods that are low in fat and contain whole-grain carbohydrates give your brain memory-enhancing glucose.
- Apples, avocados, and broccoli. These foods contain boron, which is responsible for hand-eye coordination, attention, and short-term memory. Boron-rich foods also maintain healthy bone and blood sugar levels.
- The smell of lemons can induce the feeling of alertness and they are a great alkaline food source so squeeze a quarter of a lemon on all your meals.
- Sunflower seeds contain magnesium, which helps maintain normal muscle and nerve function and keeps heart rhythm steady and bones strong. It is also involved in energy metabolism and protein synthesis. Just a handful of sunflower seeds will give you half of your daily magnesium needs.
- Tuna makes a great lunch or after-workout meal. Tuna contains the protein needed to repair muscles and supplies tyrosine for alertness.
- Salmon, or any other cold-water fish, contains the mood-elevating vitamin B12 as well as omega-3 fatty acids that may assist in preventing depression. Omega-3 raises serotonin levels in the brain. Serotonin regulates mood and reduces irritability. Eating fish to regulate your mood isn't instantaneous. It is a long-term process, and therefore, it would be beneficial to regularly incorporate fish into your diet.

- Bananas contain vitamin B6, which is known to build serotonin levels. If you regularly drink alcohol or if you are taking birth control pills, you could be depleting your body of vitamin B6. Eat your bananas with 10 to 15 almonds or add them to a smoothie.
- An amino acid called L-arginine found in nuts and sesame seeds enhances blood flow throughout your body. Eggs and meat also contain small amounts of L-arginine.
- Chocolate contains L-arginine. Yes! Everyone's favourite! This treat releases pleasure-enhancing endorphins into the brain and also contains phenylethylamine, a stimulant associated with love and sexual attraction. If you are going to eat chocolate, go for organic dark chocolate! Remember, if you have eaten 80% clean all week, then it is okay to reward yourself with a couple pieces of chocolate – but not the whole block!

Other Tips to Remember

- Break the bread-first habit. Order a chicken or tuna salad first – protein primes the brain to produce dopamine, a chemical that keeps you alert. Carbohydrates, on the other hand, cause the body to release serotonin, a calming brain chemical.
- Have at least one iron-rich food per day. Iron helps transport oxygen to your tissues, makes energy and helps boost immunity. Good sources of iron include red meats, the dark meat of chicken or turkey, beans, peas, nuts, seeds, prunes, oysters, spinach, and legumes.
- Watch your intake of alcohol and coffee. Alcohol is a sedative that can also cause dehydration. Coffee can pep you up in the

short term, but can cause you to drop like a ton of bricks later. Counter every glass of alcohol or coffee with two glasses of water.

- Try to drink at least eight glasses of water per day. Water can help to control your appetite and works as a cleansing agent for your body!

Need to Drop 2 to 3 Kilograms for a Special Occasion?

If there is a special occasion coming up, then by being a little more disciplined and strict with your nutrition, you can look fabulous!

In a nutshell, we follow these ten guidelines for two weeks to look our best:

1. Drink at least three litres of filtered water everyday
2. Cut out all fruit and sugar
3. Cut out all milk, yoghurt, cheese, cottage cheese, and ice cream
4. Do not add salt to any meals and cut out all canned and junk food. Avoid all foods with a high salt content such as pickles, smoked chicken, salted nuts, crisps, butter/margarine, tomato sauce, ketchup, thai/chinese meals, pizza, salad dressings, stock cubes, cheese.
5. Cut out alcohol
6. Eat carbohydrates at breakfast only, and lots of vegies and salads with the other meals.
7. Do 40 minutes of cardiovascular activity <u>everyday</u> – bike, run, walk, swim, kickbox, cross train

8. Do 40 minutes of fusion workouts, circuit class, or light weights <u>everyday</u>
9. Double your daily intake of green whole food supplements – spirulina and barley grass.
10. Reduce water intake on the last 2 days to only 1 litre per day.

We also use the following diuretic foods and herbs in most of our meals to help lose water weight before a main event. If you have done all the hard work in training, once you lose a bit of fluid from the body, your muscles will start to show and you will have a great lean look.

- Dandelion (tablet or tea form)
- Green tea
- Asparagus
- Parsley
- Cucumber
- Celery
- Lemon
- Garlic
- Peppermint tea

The last important thing before that special occasion, and one we use all the time, is to get a spray tan and haircut!

Chapter 18 — Mood Foods and Special Occasions

If you think you are beaten, you are,
If you think you dare not, you don't.
If you like to win, but think you can't,
It's almost a cinch you won't.

If you think you're losing, you've lost.
For out in the world we find -
Success begins with a person's will,
It's all in the state of mind.

Think big and your deeds will grow,
Think small and you'll fall behind
Think that you can and you will,
It's all in the state of mind.

If you think you're outclassed, you are,
You have to think big to rise.
You've got to be sure of yourself,
Before you can win the prize.

Life's battles don't always go,
To the strongest woman or man
But sooner or later the person who wins
Is the person who thinks they can.

—**Author Unknown**

Chapter 19

– Move It to Lose It

"Those who think they have no time for exercise will sooner or later have to find time for illness."

—**Edward Stanley,** 15th Earl of Darby

We were born to move. The human body was designed to be mobile, but due to technology and lifestyle changes, we now use wheels more than our legs to get around. Exercise is your lifeline to a healthy and fit life. It is all about developing an attitude or mindset that is action-based. Too many people associate exercise with pain and are constantly working out ways to avoid it all together. This attitude is dangerous as they do not understand the numerous benefits of exercising the body.

Chapter 19 — Move It to Lose It

You can probably come up with plenty of excuses for why you're not more active. You're too young, you're too old, you're too busy, you're too tired, or you're in pretty good shape for your age... With few exceptions, these are pretty flimsy! There are activities for the young and old, and for those with little time. So, the next time you think about getting fit, don't ask, "Who has the time?" Instead, ask yourself, "How do I make the time to feel and look better?"

Fit exercise into your day-to-day life. Monica catches up with friends all the time who have children, and they go for long walks. Monica will wear her three kilogram weighted Nikken shoes to get more of a workout and always pushes the baby stroller! There was a time when we went to Tasmania to visit family and friends, Monica had our 3-year-old niece, Stella who weighs 10 kilograms in the backpack. She was also pushing another friend's two-year-old daughter, Brylee, who weighed eight kilograms, in the pram while wearing her weighted shoes! For her it was a way to get her exercise while socializing, on holiday. For her it is just a part of life. She has exercised all her life, so to not exercise in some way, every day, would be a crime! Having Ralph, our Basenji dog helps because he must have a run outside every day or he will tear the house apart. We need to learn a lesson from our pets!

Every day take care of your body like it is your greatest asset on this planet because it is. It is your home, your house where your mind lives.

Write a list of five things you could do each day to look after your body and treat it with respect, and stick to it for a week!

Train with a partner, do a class or join a team sport – you are guaranteed to get more laughs in an exercise session with others than one on your own!

Try a dance class or new aerobics class and laugh at yourself!

Remember that exercise is not just about losing weight. It is more than that, especially when you consider the benefits of exercise:

- Reduced body fat
- Increased energy levels throughout the day
- Increased flexibility
- Injury rehabilitation
- Reduced tension and stress levels
- Beneficial effect on depression, hypochondria, and absenteeism at work
- Elevated metabolism so that you burn more calories every day – metabolism is the rate at which your body produces energy
- Increased aerobic capacity (fitness level) – this gives you the ability to go through your day with less relative energy expenditure and enables a "fit" person to have more energy at the end of the day
- Maintains, tones, and strengthens muscle, thus increasing muscular endurance
- Decreased blood pressure
- Increased oxidation (breakdown and use) of fat

Chapter 19 — Move It to Lose It

- Increased HDL (good) cholesterol
- A more efficient heart pump by increasing stroke volume
- Increased haemoglobin concentration in your blood – haemoglobin is part of the red blood cell that carries oxygen from the lungs to the rest of the body
- Decrease the tendency of the blood to clot in the blood vessels. This is important because small clots travelling in the blood are often the cause of heart attacks and strokes
- Increased bone strength
- The development of new blood vessels in the heart and other muscles
- Enlarged arteries that supply blood to the heart
- Decreased blood levels of triglycerides (fat)
- Improved control of blood sugar
- Improved sleep patterns
- Increased thickness of cartilage in joints, which has a protective effect on the joints
- Decreased risk of developing endometriosis by 50% for women
- Increased blood flows to the skin, making it look and feel healthier
- Increased efficiency of the digestive system, which may reduce the incidence of colon cancer
- Increased production of HGH in the body (human growth hormone), which is the hormone responsible for cell regeneration
- It feels great!

Exercise must become one of those things that you do without question, like bathing and brushing your teeth. Unless you are convinced of the benefits and the risks of unfitness, you will not succeed.

Since the beginning of time, survival has been a daily struggle. Simply staying alive was physically demanding. Yet, humans in industrialized societies have become spoiled over the last 150 years. We now live in our minds so much of the time that we have almost forgotten that we have a body. Many people work in offices and make their livings by reading, writing, speaking, and thinking, but seldom by physical labour.

Today there is a growing emphasis on looking good, feeling good, and living longer. Increasingly, scientific evidence tells us that one of the keys to achieving these ideals is fitness and exercise. But, if you spend your days at a sedentary job and pass your evenings as a couch potato, it may require some determination and commitment to make regular activity a part of your daily routine. You're never too unfit, too young, or too old to get started.

The key to a lifetime of fitness is consistency

- Choose an activity you enjoy.
- Tailor your program to your own fitness level.
- Set realistic goals.
- Choose an exercise that fits your lifestyle.
- Give your body a chance to adjust to your new routine.
- Don't get discouraged if you don't see immediate results.
- Don't give up if you miss a day; just get back on track the next day.

- Find a partner for a little motivation and socialization.
- Build some rest days into your exercise schedule.
- Listen to your body. If you have difficulty breathing, or experience faintness, or prolonged weakness during or after exercise, consult your physician.

Patience is essential. Don't quit before you have a chance to experience the rewards of improved fitness. You can't regain in a few days, or weeks, what you have lost in years of sedentary living, but you can get it back if you persevere – the prize is worth the price.

Physical fitness is to the human body what fine tuning is to an engine. It enables us to perform up to our potential. It gives us the ability to perform the daily tasks in our lives with vigour and alertness, and provides additional energy for enjoying leisure-time activities, and to face any emergency. Physical fitness allows us to endure stress and persevere in circumstances where an unfit person could not perform. It is the basis for good health and well-being.

Since what we do with our bodies also affects what we do with our minds, fitness influences, to some degree, such qualities as mental alertness and emotional stability.

Fitness is an individual quality that varies from person to person. It is influenced by age, gender, genetics, personal habits, exercise, and eating practices. You can't do anything about the first three factors. However, it is within your power to change and improve the others.

How often, how long, how hard you exercise, and what kinds of exercises you do should be determined by what you are trying to accomplish. Specifically, pick the right kind of activities to affect each component. Strength training results in specific strength changes. Also, train for a specific activity that you're interested in. Personally, I love cycling mainly due to the condition of my knees. It is one of the best exercises I can now do continually that is pain-free and excellent for my cardiovascular fitness. After the accident, I decided to get a top of the range bike, with front suspension, so I would never get trapped in a pot hole again. My new bike is a black Cannondale Bad Boy Ultra. I love it and ride it everywhere. Some days, I will go for a long ride, 100 to 200 kilometres, or I might do one kilometre sprints around the river. Other days, I ride hills. I mix it up to constantly shock my body so as to obtain the many associated fitness benefits. Monica loves to run with our dog Ralph, every day. When it comes to exercise, if you do what you love, and love what you do, then exercise will never be a chore for you.

Concentrate less on dropping kilograms and more on building muscle and losing fat. Muscle burns 35 calories per day while fat uses up just 3 calories per day. Make sure you are doing a resistance program three to four times a week using weights, or incorporating push-ups, sit-ups, and tricep dips into your outdoor walks, bike rides, or runs. Below are two recommendations:

- Overload – work hard enough, at levels that are vigorous and long enough to overload your body above its resting level, to bring about improvement. You can't hoard physical fitness. At least five balanced workouts a week are necessary to maintain a desirable level of fitness.

- Progression – increase the intensity, frequency, and/or duration of activity over periods of time, in order to improve.

Your body restructures, rebuilds, and regulates your hormonal responses during sleep. Sleep deprivation reduces your body's ability to deal with stress. When you struggle with stress, your body tries to help you by producing the stress hormone cortisol. Constant stress results in constant release of cortisol, which acts, along with high insulin levels, to send fat to storage at the waist.

Exercise is powerful anti-stress medicine. It improves your mood and enhances relaxation by increasing the release of endorphins for 90 to 120 minutes after a workout. To optimize exercise's anti-stress benefits, choose an activity suited to your personality.

Exercise makes us breathe better and allows more oxygen to move around our body which is very important when you look at the following study: Dr. Otto Warburg, winner of the 1931 Nobel Prize for his studies in cell respiration, believed that a person's level of health and vitality has a direct correlation to the levels of oxygen in his or her blood stream. As a test, he placed rat cells in a jar with both normal and 60% below normal oxygen levels. In the jars with lower oxygen levels, some cells weakened or died while others mutated.

—Dr Otto Warburg,
"On The Origin of Cancer Cells",
SCIENCE, (Feb, 24 1956)

Incidental Exercise

The suggestions outlined over the next few pages are a way that you can do up to one to two hours of exercise every day without even stepping into a gym or on a treadmill!

Making incidental exercise part of your everyday life is like making retirement contributions. Making a little contribution out of each pay packet won't have a significant impact on your lifestyle that week, but by retirement you will have a substantial net worth that can dramatically affect your future lifestyle.

Incidental exercise works the same way. Just by making little decisions every day to be more active, you will determine whether you spend your retirement years lying on the beach or lying in a hospital bed.

On a recent trip, Monica and I went to Byron Bay with our best friends, Brent, and Caz, who also own their own fitness centre. We went on an afternoon bushwalk. At the time they had an 18-month-old daughter, Brylee, who was in the pram. For a majority of the walk, the terrain was not suitable for the pram, so Brent and I carried it up and down mountains. It was a great workout, and we both enjoyed the challenge. Brylee stayed asleep the whole time! Along the way, Brent and I challenged each other like, "I bet you can't climb that tree in 30 seconds," or "Try to shoulder press that log 20 times!" We constantly do this wherever we go, and it makes a holiday fun. We give our bodies all the benefits of regular exercise without actually setting a specific time for it. We just include it into our life because we value it.

Chapter 19 — Move It to Lose It

We personally use all of the following incidental exercise suggestions to make sure our bodies are moving all the time. We find we sleep better and have much more energy! Try one or two of the following this week

Walk or Bike to Work Instead of Drive

Leave your car at home, or park further from work for a week, and come up with another way to get to and from work. Wear running shoes while walking to work and throw your work shoes in your bag. Putting your bike in the back of the car and parking out of city limits where there are no parking fees, saves you money and you get fit at the same time.

Exercise Before You Leave Your Bedroom

Do some stretches, or yoga, or pump out some push-ups before you leave your room in the morning. If you do them before anyone knows you are awake, then you don't have to worry about interruptions, and your whole day will be free.

Use Commercials to Exercise

Rather than sit and watch commercials, get up and move! Do housework, put clothes away, prepare your meals for tomorrow, do as many push-ups or sit-ups as you can before your show comes back. Do walking lunges up the hallway, or rent a stationary bike and ride your way through all your TV shows! Or even better, jump on your rebounder (small exercise trampoline)

Lunchtimes

Go for a 20-minute power walk first, then eat lunch. Try not to go from your desk straight into a café seat and then back to your desk! A 20-minute power walk will give you energy for the rest of the day. If you are allowed to eat at your desk, then there is no excuse not to go for a 40-minute walk or run at lunchtime then eat later! Once a week at lunchtime, try catching up with friends or colleagues for a walk or run, yoga session or fitness class at your nearest gym.

Don't Stress about Parking

Can't find a close spot at the store? Why even bother looking? Park way in the back and take the opportunity to walk. You'll save yourself some stress and burn some calories.

Take the Stairs Rather than the Lifts

Decide to never get in a lift for a whole day and walk those stairs!

Help with The Kids

Volunteer to take the kids (yours, your family's, whoever is around) to the park. Play chase with them, or throw a ball around. Offer to push the pram of your friend's children or carry the baby in the backpack! The kids will have fun, the parents will be happy, and you'll get some exercise.

Walk to the Shops for Groceries

If the store is too far to walk, park a few blocks away from the store and walk from there. If possible, don't use the trolley and carry all your groceries home or to the car.

Chapter 19 — Move It to Lose It

Take Advantage of Airport Stopovers

Flying? Walk around the airport; browse the gift shops. No reason to spend your waiting time sitting, there will be plenty of that on the plane. If you don't mind people staring, even do some yoga or stretching!

Being fit and strong through exercise gives you the ability to meet any physical or mental challenges that you may face daily.. You cannot predict what will happen in your life, so be prepared!

The consensus of the medical staff that treated me at Royal Melbourne Hospital after the accident was that if I had not been physically fit, I would have died. The main contributing factor to my survival was my high level of health and fitness.

One of the most amazing contributors, apart from initially surviving the accident, was my rate of recovery. This shocked everyone, including myself, but no one more than the transit police. On the Sunday night of the accident, the transit police were present and were witness to my injuries. On the following Friday, they came into the hospital, and I will never forget the look on their faces.

I was lying in a ward with about four other patients and they walked in, looked around the room, and walked out. Two minutes later, they walked back into the room, led by a nurse, and stood at the end of my bed with shocked faces. The female officer struggled to communicate the following words, "Are you Matt Thom?" I replied, "Yes, I am." Then there was silence for about a minute and her next words were, "I am sorry; I am a little bit jaded at the moment. I didn't expect to see you like this." I then mentioned that I was just as surprised by anyone at how quickly my body had recovered.

If you were not physically fit, do you think you could run out of a building as fast as necessary in an emergency to save your life, carry someone who is injured, deal with an accident, run from an attacker, or beat a cold or flu? Do you want to die 20 years earlier of a disease because you failed to keep fit or eat the right foods? Imagine the experiences you will miss – your grandchildren, exotic places you have never seen, exciting people to meet, and your family. You owe it to your family to live on this earth as long as you can – and the only sure way of doing this is to exercise regularly and eat a variety of healthy foods. There is no easy way out. If you do not exercise or eat well, you are lazy and need to start moving now. Choose to live today!

"Walking is man's best medicine."

—Hippocrates, c. 460-c. 377 BCE

Walking not only strengthens the muscles and bones, it's good for the heart and your digestion. Walking relaxes the mind and soothes the spirit and it doesn't cost a thing. All you need is a pair of comfortable shoes and a dog (optional).

Being fit keeps you alert, by getting the blood moving around the body and to the brain. Making decisions at work and at home becomes easier. You feel good about yourself from training hard; and that shows in your confidence – the way you walk and talk. You feel on top of the world.

Why would you choose not to exercise? Being fit is the only way to be. It is too late to say, "If only I were more fit," when a challenging event happens. There is no one to blame but yourself. It's simple – look at each day and work out all the possible times you can get your body moving! Make exercise a habit every day – just like brushing your teeth. You wouldn't miss doing that would you?

Here are some other tips on starting to exercise:

- Join a gym and try all the exciting classes they have every day – kickboxing, indoor cycling, circuit, and dance
- Get a personal trainer and be accountable for the exercise you do
- Get a big dog so that you have no choice but to walk every day
- Walk your kids to and from school
- Walk to a playground and play with your kids; don't just sit there and watch
- Weight training develops greater lean muscle mass and firms and tones the body. The more muscle you have, the more fat you burn while at rest
- Schedule your workouts each week. Make it a top priority rather than doing it only if you have time. You'll create more time in your day by the increased energy level that results from exercising, thereby allowing you to get things done more efficiently! Failing to plan is planning to fail!

As I said, Monica and I have a no excuse policy; you either do it or you don't. After 15 years of training thousands of clients, we have heard it all. At times, there may be a valid reason for not exercising at a certain time, but everyone has the same 24 hours in a day and there is ample opportunity to squeeze a minimum of 20 minutes in before you get into bed at night. Make exercise the one thing in your life that is non-negotiable. It should be a permanent part of your daily routine, like eating and sleeping. Life can be a roller coaster ride of ups and downs, and surprises at every corner; exercise keeps you resilient.

"Nothing will work unless you do!"

—John Wooden

What is the Best Exercise for a Toned, Fit Body?

So far we have talked about the benefits of exercise, its importance in relation to our health and vitality, and ways to incorporate it into your lifestyle. But what is the answer to the big million dollar question, "What is the best exercise to do that is going to give me the best results, in the shortest possible time?"

There has been a lot of research done on this question, and many books have been sold, all claiming to have a new revolutionary workout secret. It is no wonder then, that we get confused and disillusioned with exercise when there is so much conflicting information. The science of exercise is an evolving subject with many specialized areas including human performance, sport-specific training, and weight loss. This is due to advances in technology that allow us to understand more about the physiological function of the human body. There are many hypotheses and theories in these three areas. While many are in agreement, there are a few conflicting theories. What we believe to be the best and most effective way of training has come from years of research and reading countless exercise science publications, and books on exercise physiology. Initially, this knowledge was used to gain the competitive edge for us to be in the best shape of our lives and win fitness competitions. What has worked on our bodies has also worked for thousands of clients we have educated over the last decade.

> *"Fitness – if it came in a bottle, everybody would have a great body!"*
>
> —**Cher**

This is where our discussion can become a little confusing due to all the exercise terminology, but I will try to keep it simple.

Calories

"Calories, calories, calories" is what we tend to hear from food manufacturers and marketing campaigns as a buzzword to entice you to buy their products. We buy these under the assumption that low-calorie foods are better for you and eating fewer calories will cause more weight loss. In actual fact, reducing calories can do two things which can be detrimental to losing body fat.

First, reducing calories can create more stress in the body, which activates a stress hormone called cortisol. The production of cortisol releases stored sugar in the body, triggering the pancreas to release insulin. As previously mentioned too much insulin blocks fat burning. Other factors that also trigger increased insulin levels are sugar, refined carbohydrates, bottled juices, and alcohol.

Second, eating fewer calories slows down the thyroid gland, a small organ at the base of your neck which produces hormones that influence your metabolism and plays a huge part in burning fat.

Calories are simply a measure of the amount of energy provided by the food we eat. For us to decrease our body fat, we need to burn off more calories than we eat. The more calories we eat the more energy we are giving our body. However, if you don't use this energy then it is stored in the body as fat. Fat loss is nothing more than burning off more calories than we eat.

As mentioned previously in Chapter 10 Monica and I do NOT count calories in our eating plan. We never have. We just choose to eat those foods that are higher in calories, at the start of the day, so we have more energy for the activities ahead. We eat lower calorie foods, at the end of the day when we don't need the energy. So, develop the mindset that food is fuel. If you plan to get active then fill up your tank.

Metabolism

In relation to weight loss, understanding metabolism is critical. Your metabolism is the rate at which the body uses energy to support the basic functions essential to sustain life plus all energy requirements for additional activity and digestive processes. It is, quite simply, how much energy or calories your body uses per unit of time.

It takes energy to burn energy, which means you have to eat to metabolise. We must eat enough to keep all our internal systems operating at their peak performance. When it comes to losing weight, the last thing we need is for our bodies to slow down by not eating. As we speed up our metabolism, fat is burned even faster.

Metabolic rate tends to fall as we age, partly because of decreased activity. Diets can lower your metabolism, too. Very low-calorie diets, which typically restrict calories to 800 or fewer per day, slow your metabolic rate almost immediately and keep it low for weeks after the diet ends. These diets send your body into a starvation mode in which your cells try to conserve energy as much as possible by holding onto calories.

For long-term fat loss, we have to increase the speed of our metabolism, which is affected and controlled by the thyroid and is partly determined by the amount of lean tissue (muscle) we have. A good guide to follow is, the more lean tissue you have, the higher your metabolic rate. The less muscle you have, the lower your metabolic rate.

Every kilogram of muscle you put on means that you have to eat more calories per day to maintain that muscle, while at rest! Plus, there are more calories burned to move and develop the muscle. The only tissue in the body that burns fat is muscle. The more muscle we have the more fat we burn! Research also indicates that a low calorie intake can cause the body to lose a significant amount of muscle, directly suppressing metabolism by up to 45%. This is a perfect example of why we don't count calories.

We always tell our clients to never watch the scales. Always go on your body fat percentages, measurements, and clothes. One client got on the scales after six weeks of training hard, and eating a clean diet, to find she had not lost any weight at all! She came to us in tears and the first question we asked was, "Are your clothes fitting any differently?" She said, "Yes, I have dropped from a size 16 to size 12 and my old clothes no longer fit." We then did her measurements again and solved her problem: She had lost four kilograms of fat, but had put on four kilograms of muscle! She looked fantastic. Concentrate on changing the shape of your body, not dropping weight on the scales. A perfect way to lose body fat is to increase your muscle mass and increase metabolism.

Six Ways You Can Increase Your Metabolism

1. **Eat smaller meals more often** – There is scientific evidence to suggest that by eating smaller meals every three hours, rather than three large meals that are roughly five hours apart, metabolism increases. Frequent eating speeds up your metabolism because it takes energy to digest the food. More frequent eating and snacking helps to stabilize your blood sugar and gives you more energy throughout the day. If you skip breakfast, or any other meal, you are actually slowing the rate at which your body burns calories. We tell clients who do their

training at night to halve their lunch meal and eat the other half around 4:00 p.m. to give them energy for the gym after work.

2. **Eat high protein foods** – Foods such as chicken, fish, egg whites and lean red meat help to speed up the metabolism and burn more fat simply because they require so much energy for complete digestion.

3. **Spice it up** – Adding spices to your meals can increase our metabolism for up to three hours after eating. Fat-burning spicy foods such as jalapenos, chilli, and cayenne peppers can all affect your metabolism by speeding up your heart rate.

4. **Increasing antioxidants** - Our cells may progressively undergo oxidative stress as we age, and this may slow down our metabolism. Antioxidants can help fight the free radicals that are responsible for this. There are some super juices that are the highest antioxidant supplements on the market today.

5. **Supplements** – Certain supplements such as caffeine, guarana, and green tea have a thermogenic effect on the body, thus increasing metabolism. They increase the body's core temperature, increase heart rate, and help the body convert fat into lean tissue.

6. **Exercise** – The most important one of all. Getting active and moving the muscles is a sure fire way of increasing the amount of muscle you have. As stated earlier, more muscle means more calories burned, which means faster metabolism, which means you lose weight and stay fit. Doesn't it seem logical that if you don't start exercising, you will decrease your ability to burn fat? That equals slow metabolism.

What Types of Exercise Training Should I Do?

Now, let's take a closer look at the different types of exercise training and work out what activity is best for burning fat and increasing muscle. While exercising, our muscles burn fat and glucose in different proportions. Most exercises can be performed as aerobic low intensity (burns fat) or anaerobic high intensity (burns mainly carbohydrates). The terms aerobic and anaerobic simply refer to the energy system required.

Anaerobic Training

Anaerobic means "without oxygen." These exercises are high-intensity and can only be maintained for short periods. Anaerobic exercise includes sprinting, boxing, skipping, circuits, weight training, and our fitness routines. Anaerobic workouts involve quick amounts of energy, which are powered by non-oxygen fuel sources such as adenosine triphosphate and glycogen stored in the muscles. Anaerobic exercises require more effort, and up to 96% of the fuel used will be carbohydrates.

Aerobic Training

Aerobic means with oxygen. Aerobic exercises are relatively low-intensity and can be maintained for longer periods, so long as oxygen is being supplied to working muscles. Aerobic activities like walking and running are typically performed for a longer period of time. Commonly called the "fat burning zone" by many exercise specialists, this lower intensity exercise makes the body burn 50% of calories from fat while all higher intensity exercises only burn 35% calories from fat. Therefore, your body will burn a larger percentage of fat during a lower impact exercise.

Anaerobic vs. Aerobic

So, it looks like low intensity aerobic exercise may appear to be the most effective way to lose fat. BUT, aerobic cardiovascular workouts only burn fat DURING the workout. What if we told you that anaerobic workouts burn calories during, PLUS up to 24 hours AFTER, workouts? They help burn fat indirectly by increasing the body's metabolic rate, AFTER the session.

Anaerobic exercises burn more calories than aerobic exercises because each movement requires more force from the cells. Anaerobic workouts such as weight training, interval training, and circuits burn calories from carbohydrates during the workout, but the calories you burn after the exercise session are mostly calories from fat.

The ground-breaking study that illustrates the point that anaerobic high-intensity training is more effective in reducing body fat than low intensity aerobic exercise was performed by Angelo Tremblay, Ph.D., in 1994 at Laval University, Quebec, Canada. This study is outlined below.

Dr. Tremblay compared the impact of moderate-intensity aerobic exercise and high-intensity anaerobic exercise on fat loss. They divided 27 inactive, healthy, non-obese adults (13 men and 14 women, who were 18 to 32 years old), into two groups and subjected one group to a 20-week endurance training (ET) program of uninterrupted cycling four or five times a week for 30 to 45 minutes. The intensity level began at 60% of heart rate reserve (maximum heart rate minus your resting heart rate) and progressed to 85%.

The other group completed a 15-week program including mainly high-intensity-interval training (HIIT). Much like the ET group, they began with 30-minute sessions of continuous exercise at 70% of heart rate reserve, but soon progressed to 10 to 15 bouts of short (15 seconds progressing to 30 seconds) or four to five long (60 seconds progressing to 90 seconds) intervals separated by recovery periods allowing heart rate to return to 120-130 beats per minute. The intensity of the short intervals was initially fixed at 60% of the maximal work output in 10 seconds, and that of the long bouts corresponded to 70% of the individual maximum work output in 90 seconds. Intensity on both was increased 5% every three weeks.

The total energy cost of the ET program was a good deal more than the HIIT program. The researchers concluded that the ET group burned more than twice as many calories while exercising than the HIIT program. But, skin fold measurements showed that the HIIT group lost more subcutaneous fat and when the difference in the total energy cost of the program was considered, the subcutaneous fat loss was nine times greater in the HIIT program than in the ET program.

Dr. Tremblay's group took muscle biopsies and measured muscle enzyme activity to determine why high-intensity exercise produced so much more fat loss and the result proved that compared to moderate-intensity endurance exercise, high-intensity intermittent exercise causes more calories and fat to be burned after the workout.

Reference: Tremblay, A., J. Simoneau, and C. Bouchard. "Impact of Exercise Intensity on Body Fatness and Skeletal Muscle Metabolism." Metabolism, 43:814-818, 1994.

Shocking the Body to Drop Fat

The human body is a survival machine. Its primary job is to keep us alive, and, at times, we can make this job very difficult. The body deals with change every day, constantly adapting to our environment, the food we eat, the way we move, as well as millions of biochemistry changes on a cellular level that we aren't even aware of. It does this to keep us at a point of balance for optimum function. For example, when you are frightened, your body releases adrenalin, known as the fight or flight response. The adrenalin is there to help you survive that particular situation. If you stopped drinking water, then your body would retain more fluid. So when you decide to go on a diet and start an exercise regime, you start seeing some good results until your body adapts to the decreased calories and slows down the metabolism. Your body can get used to aerobic exercise within a period of four to six weeks. Have you ever wondered why you see so many aerobic instructors that take up to 10 classes a week, but are still overweight? It is because their bodies have adapted to this level of activity and responded by slowing metabolism and storing fat.

When we work out with resistance, like weight training, we are actually tearing muscle fibres and breaking down muscle tissue, which is called atrophy. The body adapts to this by building more lean tissue.

Another reason why anaerobic exercise is so much better than aerobic exercise for changing the shape of your body is adaptation. The biggest problem with aerobic training is that your body gets used to it and you get better at it. To improve, you must run, walk, or bike longer or faster to burn the same number of calories. Eventually, the new speed becomes too easy for you, and you have to become more intense to get the same benefit. You start to see the finish line with your aerobic training and need an extra boost.

The good news with anaerobic weight circuit training is that there is *no* end! When you get better in weight training and circuit work, you can add more weight, do more repetitions, or increase the intensity. The exercises for anaerobic training are limitless.

Resistance Training

Resistance training puts a load on the muscles and makes them work really hard. Weight machines, dumbbells, and barbells are the classic choices of equipment when it comes to resistance training. With the right program, and correct technique, it is a sure fire way to increase the amount of muscle in your body, which, as discussed, has many benefits. Remember:

- Muscle is the only tissue that burns fat
- Muscle requires more calories for movement
- Muscle increases metabolism
- For hours after resistance training, muscles burn more calories from fat

We recommend resistance training *at least* two days per week – one day for upper body, one day for lower body. You don't have to go to a gym to do resistance training. When we travel, we always take our trusty gym stick. It is a small, light, compact resistance training tool that we have used in hotel rooms, at parks, on beaches, and in the lounge room.

Resistance training is crucial, and when you are busy or travelling, a gym stick allows you to get a hard, phenomenal workout anywhere! Anyone can use it, and it comes with a comprehensive DVD and training website. There are literally hundreds of exercises you can do for the whole body.

Our Fusion Workout

Taking all this information into account, whenever you do a scheduled workout, which we recommend you do at least three a week, what should you be doing? The workout we prescribe to our clients, and which we do ourselves three times a week, is what we have named the *Fusion Workout*. The Fusion Workout can work for anyone regardless of age and fitness level. It is all about personal best training. It can be adapted anywhere regardless of equipment or the environment. As the name suggests, Fusion workouts combine multiple principles of training such as strength, muscular endurance, power, and cardiovascular exercise in one intense, short, sharp session. Fusion workouts also incorporate anaerobic and aerobic training, which is also known, in the fitness industry, as High Intensity Interval Training (HIIT).

Interval training is arguably the most effective method for increasing your fitness. It involves higher interval intensity training (anaerobic) for a short period followed by short intervals of lower intensity (aerobic) exercise. Interval training can burn more calories in a shorter period of time than a continuous moderate intensity training session such as a long run, known also as *steady state training*. Your body adapts to the steady state aerobic training, whereas the beauty of interval training is that as you improve, the work intervals can get harder and the recovery periods can be shortened or done at a higher speed. There is no finish line and your body will never adapt to the training because it is constantly changing to your fitness levels – this is perfect for fat loss and achieving the body you want.

Our Fusion workouts are effective because they involve resistance training to build lean muscle and interval training to increase fitness and ultimately burn body fat. Fusion workouts are fantastic, as they cater for beginners right through to advanced athletes. We have beginner, intermediate, and advanced options in all the workouts.

How to do the Fusion Workout

We offer lots of different Fusion workouts that are each 40 to 60 minutes long in our *84 Day Body Challenge Action Manual* – all complete with colour photos and are very easy to follow.

A breakdown of the 40 to 60 minute workout looks like this:

5 minutes	Aerobic warm up
15-30 minutes	High intensity resistance circuit Two minute aerobic after each circuit completed
15-20 minutes	Interval aerobic training
5 minutes	Stretch

The five minute aerobic warm up may be any of the following: rowing, walking (flat or incline), biking, cross training, running, stairs, star jumps, high knee running, skipping.

Then we move onto a high intensity resistance circuit using our body weight, resistance bands (gym sticks), dumbbells, barbells, or machines, setting up a full-body circuit. The purpose of the resistance circuit is to overload and fatigue all muscle groups with high intensity.

The best way to incorporate a weight or exercise program into your life that is right for you is to consult a personal trainer. That way they can show you the correct lifting techniques and go over exercise safety precautions. The last thing you want is an injury, so please consult a qualified health professional. Just take the 84 Day Body Challenge Action Manual in with you.

Examples of a circuit in a Fusion workout may be:

Exercise Do 10-40 reps	Beginner	Intermediate	Advanced
Push-ups	Knee push-ups	Toe push-ups	Decline push-ups
Squats	Sumo squats	Pulsing squats	Jumping squats
Tricep dips	Bent-knee tricep dips	Straight-leg tricep dips	Heels-on-fit-ball tricep dips
Crunches	Knees bent	Lower legs at same tine	V-snap sit-ups
Chin-ups	Lying down chin-ups	Feet on fit ball chin-ups	Chin-ups on bar/ledge
Lunges	Stationery lunges	Alternating lunges	Jumping lunges

All the Fusion workouts are different and incorporate dumbbells, medicine ball, Gym Sticks, and barbells. Immediately after doing one of the circuits, move into a two-minute intense aerobic exercise. This allows the muscles to recover before we get back into the resistance circuit again. Depending on your fitness, repeat the circuit 2 to 12 times, but for no longer than 30 minutes with high intensity.

When the circuit is finished, after a maximum of 30 minutes, move onto an aerobic activity for interval training. Interval training refers to a series of intense exercises separated by short rest periods. This allows you to exercise at high intensity without getting too tired. Because we alternate between periods of high intensity work and low intensity work, you are able to do much more work (and burn more calories) in the same time period than if you were going for a 20-minute power walk or riding the bike for 20 minutes.

The next part of the Fusion workout – interval training – involves alternating high-intensity exercise with low-intensity recovery periods for 15-20 minutes. Depending on your fitness levels, start with smaller intervals and double the rest. For example, bike sprints – 10 seconds on, 20 seconds off, one minute on, two minutes off. Once you have reached a rest period of two minutes, go back to the start and match the rest with the interval period, for example, bike sprints – 10 seconds on, 10 seconds off, 30 seconds on, 30 seconds off, one minute on, one minute off.

Interval training can be done on any cardiovascular machine and outside with activities like boxing, cycling, running and skipping. Please remember, though, that if you don't feel completely recovered at the end of the recovery periods, extend them as long as you need. Your heart rate is a good guide to know when you've recovered. To finish the Fusion workout, use a five minute cool-down exercise such as walking, low intensity biking, or cross training, and then be sure to do a stretch. Refer to the *Action Manual* for a complete list of stretches with photos.

Even though you may have favourite Fusion workouts (there are 19 to choose from), keep mixing them up, at least every four weeks, to keep shocking your body and keep your metabolism firing.

Chapter 19 — Move It to Lose It

How to Turn Your Current Workouts into a Fusion Workout

Power walking with friends	Stop every 10 minutes and do as many sit-ups, push-ups, triceps dips and lunges as you can. Repeat. Find a place to walk that involves hills to tone the legs and raise your heart rate. Even try and run up the hill as far as you can. Wear leg weights on your ankles to tone up.
Riding a bike	Sprint as fast as you can, for one minute, slow down for one minute, and repeat. Do this for 30 minutes. Do a hill program on a stationary bike or find a hill outside to ride up. Get off your bike every 10 minutes and do as many sit-ups, push-ups, tricep dips, and lunges as you can. Then get back on and repeat.
Weight training only	Every eight minutes, do a hard cardiovascular blitz for two minutes such as skipping non-stop, running on an incline, hill bike riding without sitting on the seat, shuttle runs, and then return to weights.
Walking the dog	Walk for 10 minutes to an off lead park, then find an area to set up the following circuit (your dog can still run around): 10 push-ups, 10 sit-ups, 10 triceps dips, 10 lunges for each leg, and 10 burpees. Do this mini-circuit as many times as you can in 10 minutes, and then keep walking – repeat.
Running outside	Do a five minute warm up, then run as hard as you can for one minute, slow jog for two minutes, and keep repeating for 40 minutes. OR do a 10 minute run then 10 push-ups, 10 sit-ups, 10 triceps dips, 10 lunges for each leg, and 10 burpees. Do this mini-circuit as many times as you can in 10 minutes, then back into your run and keep repeating.

To make your body the ultimate fat burning machine you must do a mix of aerobic (cardiovascular) and anaerobic (weight training/circuit) exercises in three of your training sessions, using our Fusion workout.

It is very important to realise that we all need aerobic training; you can not just do anaerobic (weights). Aerobic has its own set of important functional benefits including general fitness, elastic arteries, increased heart and lung function, and lower blood pressure. So, a long run, walk, swim, or bike ride is important in your weekly training.

Did you know that exercise can help you grow brain cells? The University of Queensland's Janet Wiles, cognitive scientist and author of *The Memory Book: Everyday Habits for a Healthy Memory,* says, "Deep in the brain there's a region called the hippocampus. Most of the brain doesn't get new brain cells, but this region does. If you exercise, you get more brain cells, but if you don't use them, most will die." Physical exercise generates more new cells and mental exercise keeps them alive.

Other Feel Good Exercises to Include Every Day

Yoga

The benefits of yoga are endless. It strengthens, stretches, tones, and lengthens your body for a slim look. It improves the circulation of blood, it massages the internal organs, it facilitates inner calm and alleviates stress, it helps with injury prevention, and it gives you a more positive and balanced outlook on the world. There are many different varieties of yoga – ashtanga, iyengar, power, bikram, flow – and they are all great!

Here is a quick summary of yoga postures used in classes and all their benefits:

- Forward bends – calms the nervous system and refreshes the brain
- Twisting – cleanses and tone internal organs, improving digestion, eliminating sluggishness as well as relieving backaches, headaches, and stiff necks and shoulders
- Restorative postures – conserves and restores energy, improves circulation and respiration
- Sitting poses – energizes the body by stimulating digestion, promotes strength and flexibility in the back, hips, knees, neck, and shoulders
- Balancing poses – develops muscle tone, balance, strength, and agility
- Inverted poses and arm balances – revitalizes the entire body, improves circulation, promote balance, and mental clarity

Monica completed her yoga teaching diploma in 2003 and has been doing yoga for years, but I only started in 2006 and now do a yoga class every week. It is a great recovery session for me and gives me time to unwind.

Rebounding

We have used a rebounder (mini-trampoline) for the last six months with amazing results. We jump for five to ten minutes at a time for an energy boost, always first thing in the morning to wake the whole body. It gives your body a real *buzz*. It is also great for anyone with knee injuries because it builds up strength in the legs. A rebounder stimulates every cell in the body simultaneously. It stimulates and strengthens the immune system and is incredibly effective at cleansing toxins out of cells. It promotes and stimulates all major organs and glands, and dramatically strengthens and tones the muscles, tendons, and ligaments. Purifying the lymphatic system is vital for ridding your body of cellulite. One of the best ways to cleanse your lymphatic system is by bouncing!

Our Workout Week

If you are prepared and you have a plan then you can succeed. The following is an example of our workout week.

Day	Matt's Workouts	Monica's Workouts
Monday	Five minutes rebounding Fusion workout (morning) Weights – chest (afternoon)	40 minutes walking the dog (morning) Fusion workout (afternoon)
Tuesday	Five minutes rebounding 45 minutes Bike Ride (morning) Weights – back (afternoon)	One hour of personal training (weights, boxing) 40 minutes walk the dog (afternoon)
Wednesday	Five minutes rebounding Fusion Workout (morning) Weights – legs (afternoon) One hour yoga class (night)	40 minutes run with the dog (morning) 45 minutes kickbox/acrobatics (afternoon) One hour yoga class (night)
Thursday	Five minutes rebounding Weights – shoulders (afternoon)	40 minutes walking the dog (morning) Fusion workout (afternoon)
Friday	Five minutes rebounding Kickboxing workout (morning) Weights – arms (afternoon)	40 minutes running with the dog (morning) Fusion Workout (afternoon)
Saturday	60 minute, or more, bike ride	One hour Gym Stick Class (morning) One hour walking the dog (afternoon)
Sunday	REST	40 minutes walking the dog (morning) Yoga class (afternoon)

Chapter 19 — Move It to Lose It

Matt after Train Accident February 2001

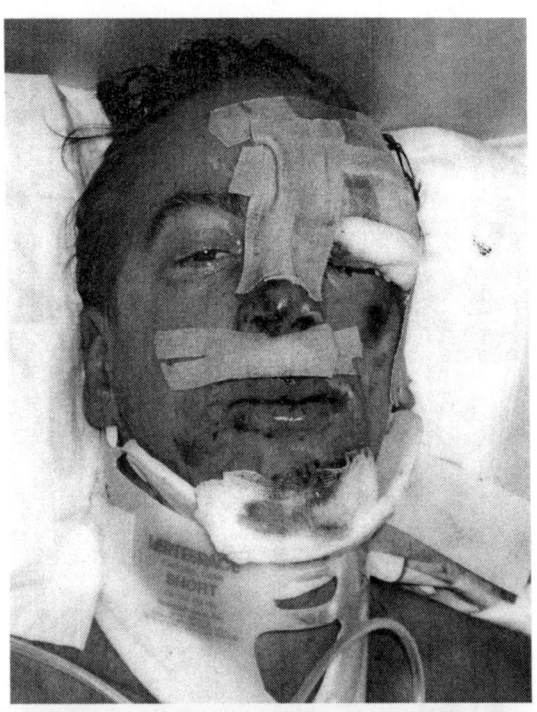

Matt with his sister in Hospital, February 2001

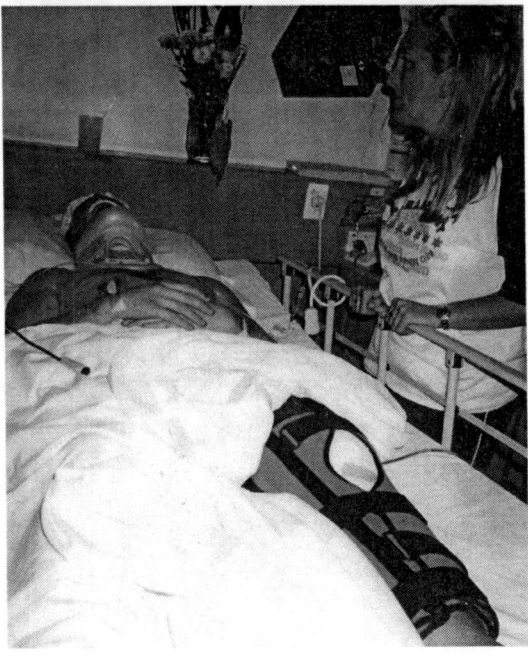

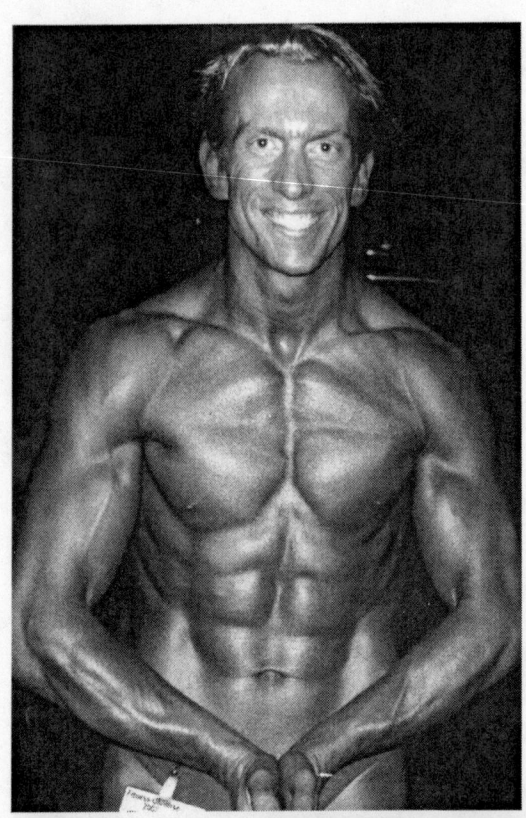

Change Your Body with the World's Fittest Couple

Winning Form in 2002

Matrix Routine at Fitness Universe 2005

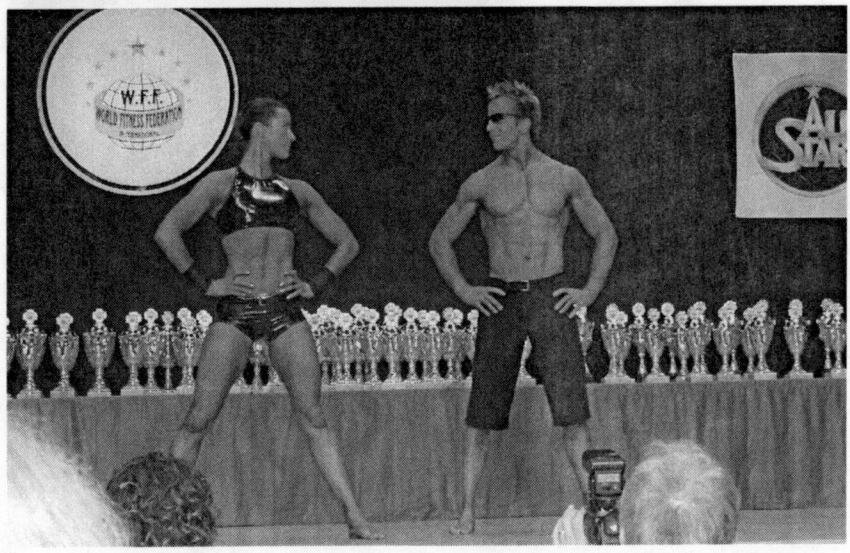

Chapter 19 — Move It to Lose It

Monica doing her fitness 'wonder woman' routine in Vegas

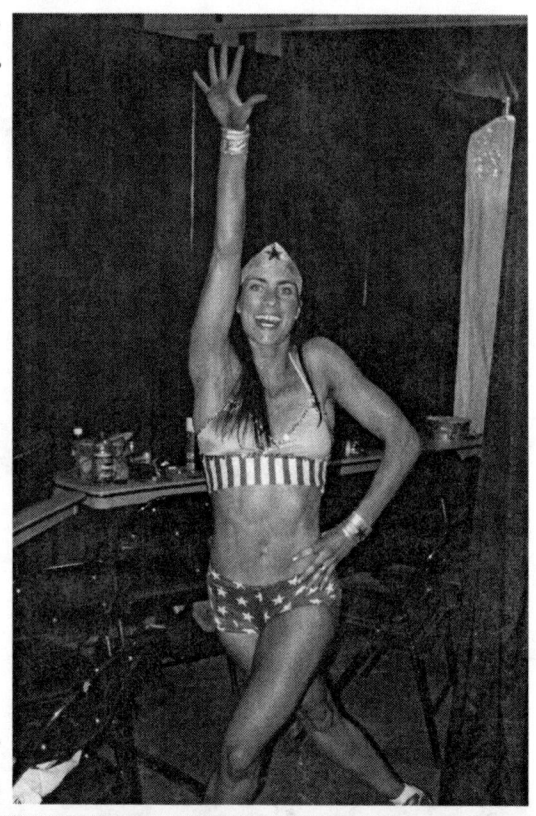

'Rocksliding' together in 2003

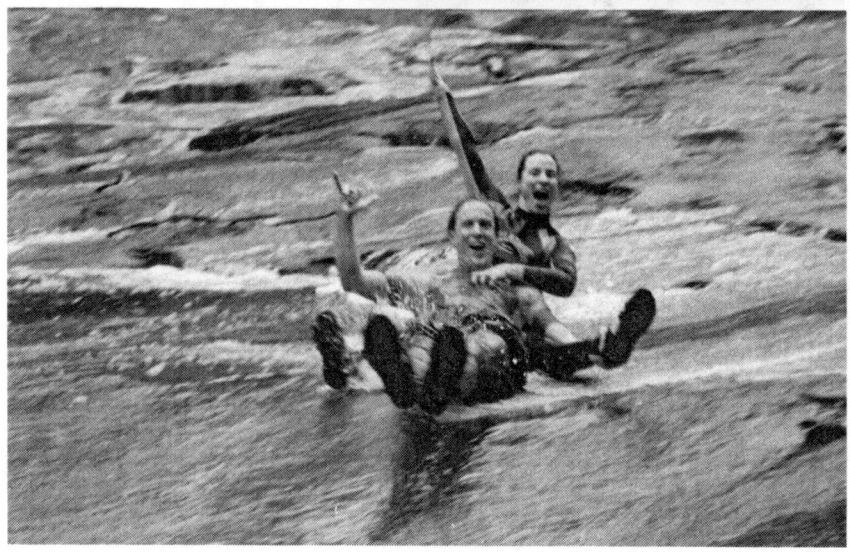

267

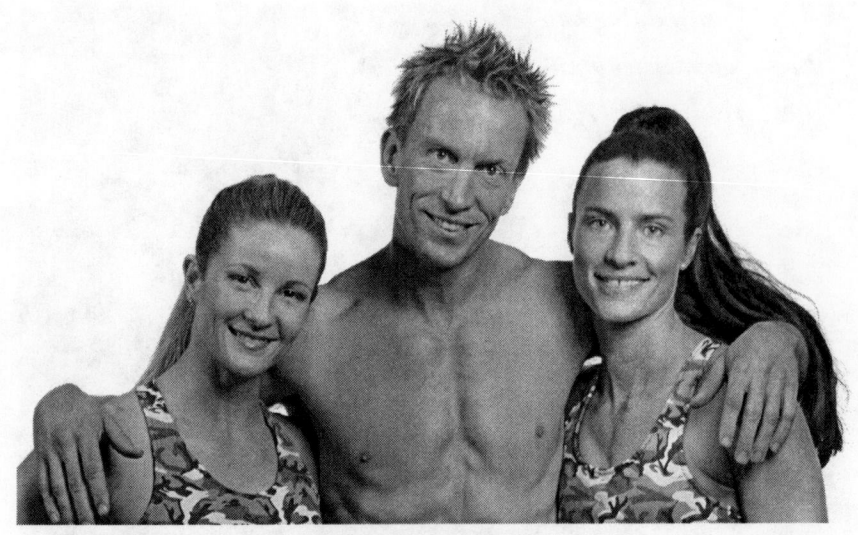

Change Your Body with the World's Fittest Couple

Matt with Ms Fitness Australia – Kerry Lugg and 4 time Ms Fitness Universe - Monica

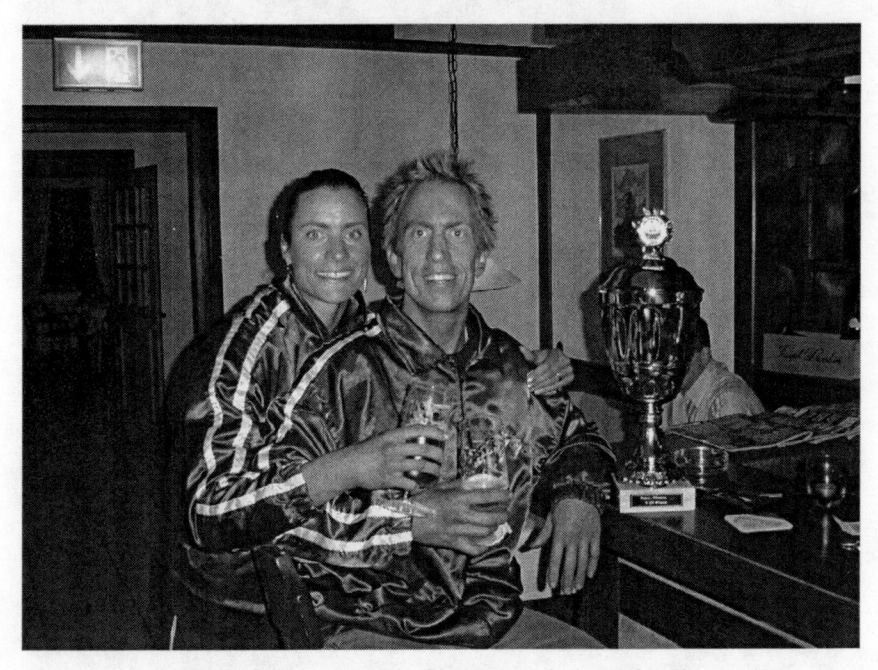

Celebration Beers after our 4th world title!

SECTION 3
STAY DEDICATED

Chapter 20

– Think Fit

LIFE IS A UNIVERSITY

A wise man once said that God gave man two ends – one to sit on and one to think with. It has been evident ever since that the success and failure of any individual was dependent on the one end he used most. Unfortunately, too many people today are sitting on their rear ends, not realizing that the way they think causes their problems. They have to straighten out the way they think if they are to improve their quality of life and achieve all of their dreams.

How do you straighten out the way you think? First, you must all realise that life is a university. The university has an infinite number of lessons and curricula that are mandatory. Of course, you can choose to skip certain classes and never reach your full potential and achieve all you were meant to. If you try and cheat on the tests or copy other people's homework, you are guaranteed an F.

But if you choose to go to class every day, take notes, study, and put the principals into action, then you will succeed and achieve all you have ever dreamed.

—Author Unknown

In this chapter, we have gone into great detail to explain the power of the mind and the subconscious. We go back and explain some areas that we have already touched on in greater depth, like visualisation and affirmations. This section attempts to get you to delve deeper inside so you can identify anything that may be holding you back that you may or may not be aware of. We also help you identify strengths that you can draw upon to help you in the future.

Every personal development book we have ever read, and every seminar we have attended, have all concluded that the single most important ingredient to any human accomplishment is the way you THINK.

When you combine exercise, clean eating, and supplements with positive affirmations, you are creating an atmosphere in your mind where anything is possible, without limits. Do you realise that every thought you think, every word you say, is an affirmation?

What's the psychological difference between healthy and unhealthy people? The difference is attributed to how they view their lives, and what they say to themselves. A lot of outcomes are predetermined by your beliefs, and your beliefs are influenced by your vision and your self-talk.

Affirmations are all of your self-talk, or inner dialogue. You are constantly affirming, subconsciously, with your words and thoughts, and this flow of affirmations is affecting your health. Since the majority of your beliefs are just learned thought patterns, you need to be acutely conscious about what you tell yourself.

This inner dialogue can be dysfunctional and may be sabotaging you from getting fit. Every affirmation you think or say is a reflection of your inner truths or beliefs. It is important to realise that many of these *inner truths* may not actually be true for you now or may be based on invalid impressions you developed as a child, which if examined as an adult, can be exposed as incorrect.

> *It takes both rain and sunshine to make a rainbow.*
>
> —**Author Unknown**

Positive affirmations are designed to challenge all of your negative beliefs. Affirmations aren't just statements repeated over and over. They are a process of becoming aware of your thoughts and words in everyday life, and of changing negative thoughts into happy and productive thoughts.

Your subconscious uses the behaviour patterns you have learned to instantly respond and react to many events in your life. This is especially true for your health. Your learned responses, and thought patterns, allow you to automatically respond to circumstances. This automatic response can be inappropriate, if at some time during your past, your belief system formed a skewed perspective regarding your true self. More often than not, your beliefs aren't aligned so that you can be healthy and live up to your fullest potential; something holds you back.

Using positive affirmations will help you to undermine and replace false beliefs with positive and self-nurturing beliefs. Positive affirmations are usually short, positive statements you repeat. The concept is quite simple. By filling your mind with negative talk, you are sabotaging your view of your health with self-deprecating doubt. On the other hand, by filling your mind with positive dialogue, you have a beautiful, abundant life, bursting with positive and creative energy.

These statements must be worded very carefully. Remember that everything you say and think can be a positive affirmation. The more determined you are to make, and accept change, the better positive affirmations will work for you. Positive affirmation statements help you to define the healthy life you've always desired.

Repeating self-affirmations creates a deep, lasting impression in your subconscious mind; the more repetitions, the deeper the impression. The following are a few guidelines for creating positive affirmations:

- Keep your affirmations as concise and specific as possible.
- Only use positive statements. Avoid words such as can't, won't, not, etc.
- Keep your affirmations in the present tense.

Start by taking some time to think about areas of your health you would like to improve and how you might want your life to be. Get a blank piece of paper and list the most important ones. After you've written them, write out a couple of positive statements for each. Remember to concentrate on what you want to improve, not what you don't want to improve. When we are in training mode for a competition, the workouts are crucial to develop the body and gain the strength required for the routine. The workouts must be done with full intensity, without question. When you combine dieting and working 60 hours a week, it can all come down to the mind game inside your head. There are some days when we have not slept well, got up early, and worked all day. When 9:00 p.m. hits, it is workout time! When you are tired and fatigued, the self-talk that starts in your head is:

- "I am too tired to work out"
- "I can't be bothered; I just want to go home to bed"
- "If I go home now, I will work harder tomorrow"

Affirmations make all the difference because they help you win the mind games. When we have a negative thought , we start exercising and repeat one of the following over and over:

- "If I work out I win."
- "The harder I train, the harder I look."
- "The very best, train the best."
- "Winners work and losers whine."
- "Every workout I get stronger and stronger."
- "If I train hard, I am hard to beat."

- "To win, you have to put in."
- "This is a workout that a winner would do, and I am a winner."

Now that you've planted your affirmations in your mind, it is time to visualise them. Your subconscious mind thinks in terms of pictures. Creating pictures allows you to take a shortcut directly into your subconscious. Visualisation creates a belief that can alter the circumstances of your life. Through visualisation, you can deliver direct messages right into your subconscious mind.

> *"You are never too old to set another goal or to dream a new dream."*
>
> —C. S. Lewis

Your subconscious mind does not have the ability to rationalize. Whatever you tell your subconscious mind, it takes as truth. So, in essence, if you consistently picture yourself as having already achieved the highest level of health, your subconscious mind will soon believe that to be true. Your subconscious must balance your inner and outer reality, and in order to do so, it sets into motion any circumstances necessary to create in the physical realm that which you believe to be true. Forcing your subconscious to accept your desire for good health, and believing it, will turn your desire into a reality.

You can visualise virtually anywhere, but a quiet, safe place where you will not be disturbed is best. Focus your mind on what you want to do, and keep replaying the internal film of yourself actually doing it. The amazing thing is that it has been proven that the benefit of visualizing the events is actually the same as if you had actually done it!

Think of how you want your health to be, concentrate, and imagine yourself in the situation, be realistic about the experience, keep it true to how you expect it to be, see yourself feeling great, everything right, imagine yourself through others eyes, seeing yourself succeed.

An effective visualisation happens when you make the images in your mind real. Think of them as movies, constantly playing in your mind. Fill your visualisations with emotion and energy. The more realistic they appear to you, the more they are becoming a reality.

Affirmations and visualisations, when combined, are powerful tools that will help you create a belief and hold a vision that will lead you to the best health of your life. Visualise your affirmations as living pictures of truth. Use affirmations and visualisations together to visualise your good health, while you repeat an affirmation for it.

> *"Get excited and enthusiastic about your own dream. This excitement is like a forest fire – you can smell it, taste it, and see it from a mile away."*
>
> **—Denis Waitley**

Chapter 20 — Think Fit

Create a picture in your mind where you see yourself achieving good health. Use short, positive statements affirming that your purpose is reality. In this way you can begin to create the reality you desire. Use the suggestions below to help you harness the power for affirmations and visualisations:

- Use as many senses as possible in affirmations and visualisations. Verbalize statements out loud after writing them down. Listen to yourself say these statements while standing in front of a mirror. When you visualise your health, recreate as much of the scene as possible to create an accurate simulation. Imagine what it sounds like, what it feels like, smells like, etc..

- Make affirmations and visualisations emotional. Imagine what it will feel like to be healthy, young, and self-assured. Visualise yourself experiencing these emotions. At the same time, work to eliminate statements of negative emotions from your life, e.g., I'm tired, I'm fat, I'm old, I'm bored.

To effectively harness the power of affirmations and visualisations, you must remove as much stress as possible from your life. For many of us, stress relief seems impossible. There is so much to deal with in our everyday lives that it seems that no end is ever in sight. The trick to stress relief is not the amount of stress you have, but how you handle it. There are many ways to reduce tension and relax.

Seven Stress Relievers You Can Start Today

The following seven stress relievers are very effective for the amount of work and time involved. Some can be learned in the time it takes to read this page, while others take a little more practice. There's something here for everyone. Find which ones help you through your day and practice them regularly.

1. Breathing Exercises

Deep breathing is an easy stress reliever that has numerous benefits for the body, including oxygenating the blood to wake up the brain, relax muscles and quiet the mind. Breathing exercises are especially helpful because you can do them anywhere, and they work quickly so you can de-stress in a flash. When was the last time you took a really deep breath? Most people have a very shallow breathing pattern, and incorrect breathing can add to your everyday stress. One way to relax under pressure and to energize the body is to purposely slow down your breathing and take long, deep breaths. In addition to feeling more energized, this type of breathing has a cleansing effect on the body. Deep breathing sends fresh oxygen around the body and promotes the removal of stagnant toxins. You can do it sitting in your car, at your desk, or lying in a park. We call it the Triple Four Breath and we use it every day. It goes like this:

- Inhale slowly for a count of four
- Hold the breath in for a count of four
- Exhale slowly for a count of four
- REPEAT!

2. Meditation.

Meditation builds on deep breathing, and takes it a step further. When you meditate, your brain enters an area of functioning that's similar to sleep. Meditation carries some added benefits you can't achieve in any other state, including the release of certain hormones that promote health. Also, the mental focus on nothingness brings your mind from working overtime and reducing stress level.

3. Massage

Your sense of touch is closely linked to your state of mind and is vital to your sense of well-being. Get a massage from a friend or a professional. If neither is available, you can use a self-massager, which will also work great in promoting circulation, releasing tension, and helping you feel more relaxed. On a recent holiday to Thailand, Monica completed a diploma in Thai Massage – how lucky am I?

4. Progressive Muscle Relaxation

By tensing and relaxing all the muscle groups in your body, you can relieve tension and feel much more relaxed in minutes, with no special training or equipment. Start by tensing all the muscles in your face, holding a tight grimace for ten seconds, then completely relaxing for ten seconds. Repeat this with your neck, followed by your shoulders, and so on. You can do this anywhere. I do it every night in the shower to relax and unwind. As you practice, you will find you can relax more quickly and easily, reducing tension as quickly as it starts!

5. Sex.

You probably already know that sex is a great tension reliever, but have you officially thought of it as a stress-relieving practice? Perhaps you could. The physical benefits of sex are numerous, and most of them work very well toward relieving stress. Sadly, many people have less sex when their stress levels are high.

6. Music.

Music therapy has shown numerous positive benefits for people with health conditions, especially stress. When dealing with stress, the right music can actually lower your blood pressure, relax your body, and calm your mind. Everyone has their own taste in music, whether it be the tranquil sounds of the ocean, top 40, or classical music. Whatever music helps you unwind, place it in your car, on your iPod, or at home. Walking while listening to music is a great combination.

7. Yoga

One of the oldest self-improvement practices, dating back over 5,000 years! It combines the practices of several other stress management techniques such as breathing, meditation, imagery, and movement, giving you a lot of benefit for the amount of time and energy required. Learn more about how to manage stress with yoga.

Now you certainly don't have to do all of these seven techniques. They have been outlined so you can choose the ones that appeal to you. For instance, sex, massage, and music are my top three!

As outlined earlier, stress is a huge reason for the body to be acidic, which consequently causes it to hold onto body fat.

In the lead up to a competition we regularly test our pH. Even though we are on the same exercise and eating plan, our pH will vary. Monica will be extremely alkaline and I will be acidic. The reason for this is that I tend to get more stressed than Monica. These stress relieving techniques are an integral part of my competition preparation and daily life.

No matter who you are or what your level of fitness is, affirmations and visualisations will improve your life. If used correctly, they can change the way you think, reprogram your mind, and remove old negative beliefs that have sabotaged your health throughout your life. You will achieve the health you've always wanted.

You cannot plough a field by turning it over in your mind.

—**Author Unknown**

To truly be fit, you must think fit. The only limitations are the ones you create in your mind. We touched on this topic briefly in previous chapters, but we would like to talk about the importance of combining the physical aspect of fitness with the mental.

A paradigm is a pattern of thought which represents the held beliefs of a person or a group of people. For the majority of us, these beliefs are negative and self-defeating. Each one of us grows up with certain beliefs about who we are and carry them with us into adulthood. Our personalities and identities were formed when we were children. Many of these beliefs aren't true, but since we accepted them at such an early age we didn't have the ability to question whether they were correct or not – we just accepted them. Ask yourself if you've experienced any of the things below:

- Certain behaviours constantly creep back into your life no matter what you do.
- You can't control your anger.
- Mistakes aren't allowed in your life.
- You are unhappy and you don't know why.
- You always compare your relationships to others, wishing they were better.
- You tell yourself, almost on a daily basis, that if only you could lose weight, then your life would be better.
- No matter what you do in life, you feel unfulfilled.

If you can relate to any of these statements, your negative beliefs are more than likely affecting your life, without you even knowing it. You are doing this subconsciously. Your life is impacted by your subconscious. Your subconscious instructs you on how to act, and react, to the events and people in your life. Unfortunately, these instructions don't match what is actually happening around you. Your subconscious can't tell time.

Your subconscious alters your past experiences into an unrealistic view to help you avoid any pain from past events in your life. This view that you have creates an unrealistic version of how your life should be, not how it actually is. Your reality becomes ingrained with this unrealistic view. A lot of work is needed to keep up with this distorted view that your subconscious has created. So what does this mean? How do you recognise when your subconscious is sabotaging you? How do you keep your subconscious from controlling every aspect of your life?

You know it is controlling you when this unrealistic view interferes with your life by causing emotional and physical pain leading to an unhealthy life. When your life is in total chaos, it is time to take an honest look at yourself. The key to understanding how this view is adversely affecting your life is to find out where this view came from. Uncovering your past beliefs is crucial. In order to uncover any of these beliefs, you have to find some of the origins of your past beliefs.

"If you want your life to be a magnificent story, then begin by realizing that you are the author and every day you have the opportunity to write a new page."

—**Mark Houlahan**

As children, your mum and dad are your world. You depended on them to give you emotional support and love. From your earliest moments, interactions with them determine what kind of person you will become, and consequently, what kind of self-image you will have. Did one of your parents reward you with junk food? Perhaps as an adult you may reward any accomplishment with a dinner at a nice restaurant or a trip to the bakery? Did you ever eat to escape the feelings of abandonment or shame?

These reactions were automatic, and you had no idea why you were doing them because it happened on a subconscious level. You are caught in a cycle. Because these subconscious thoughts begin at such an early age, your distorted view of reality becomes the basis for every future experience. You don't need this as an adult, but your subconscious won't let it go. So, you hold on to it, still believe it, and let it get in the way of your health. It is important to uncover the source so you can stop relying on your childlike responses and make positive, healthy decisions. By doing this you create a paradigm shift.

Journaling is very important in determining what experiences caused this unrealistic view about your self-image, weight, or any other aspect of your health. Writing down your false beliefs in a diary or a note book will bring them to your awareness. If you don't consciously admit your problems, they can't be acknowledged and corrected.

> *"Don't let the best you have done so far be the standard for the rest of your life."*
>
> —**Gustavus F. Swift,** 1839-1903

Start writing your thoughts on the following topics:

- What are my beliefs about my body, looks, and health?
- Where do they come from? Family? Friends? Teachers?
- How do I change these beliefs?
- What will my results be if I change a belief?
- How will my overall good health positively affect my life?

Please be patient and continue journaling even if you are feeling uncomfortable or anxious. This is the only way you can get a realistic look at which areas of your life are keeping you from becoming fit and healthy. It will also become evident what you can change (diet, activities, etc.) and what you can't (family, friends, and co-workers). Once you understand these perceptions and where they originate, you will be able move beyond them and embrace a life filled with health, energy, and love.

Unrealistic views are everywhere in your life. Maybe they came from something you were told over and over when you were a child. We hear many examples in our personal training, like:

- "There's always going to be someone more fit"
- "I am just destined to be the fat person at the office!"
- "Exercise is hard!"
- "I have to work too hard to have a body like that!"
- "I'm just not good enough!"
- "I'll never be able to lose that much weight!"
- "That's just not something I'll ever be able to do"

- "I can't quit eating junk food and drinking soft drinks"
- "I have been big my whole life"
- "My whole family is fat; it is in my genes"
- "I hardly eat anything, and I am still fat"
- "I train so hard and I don't lose anything"

"Set your sights high
The higher the better
Expect the most wonderful things to happen
Not in the future but right now
Realise that nothing is too good
Allow absolutely nothing to hamper you
Or hold you up in any way"

—**Eileen Caddy**

The Law of Attraction

What you believe, you will attract. This Universal Law is working in your life right now, whether you are aware of it or not. You are attracting the people, situations, jobs, and much more into your life. Once you are aware of this law and how it works, you can start to use it to deliberately attract what you want into your life.

How do you create your desires using this powerful law? There are just a few basic steps.

- Get very clear on what you want.
- Visualise and raise your vibration about it.
- Allow it.
- Take inspired action.

You must be very clear on exactly what you desire. **Focus on it.** Give it all your positive energy. Feel good!

Any thought you may have, when combined with emotion, vibrates out from you to the universe, and will attract what you focus on, and bring it back to you.

You can leave all the details to the universe. Let the universe figure out the method of delivery, when you will receive it, and how it will manifest itself. Now, all you have to do is allow it. Sounds easy, right? This can be the most difficult part to do. Be doubt-free. All you need to do is expect it. Act like you already have it. Be grateful.

Now take inspired action. If something feels right, then go ahead and do it. Taking action is an important step. That is it! You can always be expectant of good things and feel good knowing your desire is on its way to you. Expect miracles.

"This is your life, not a dress rehearsal."

—**John Donovan**

Be grateful! The most powerful way to use the Law of Attraction is to be grateful! Why? Because gratitude is the quickest vehicle to change your level of vibration! Simply find something to be grateful for to help you develop the right self-talk, like:

- "I am so happy now that I am..."
- "I am so grateful that I have..."
- "I love the fact that..."
- "I am so grateful that I am in the process of..."
- "I am so happy now that I choose to..."

If you feel any tension as you state your affirmations aloud, or while writing them down, you can add:

- "... and, I release any need to feel like I don't deserve this."
- "... and, I release any need to hold onto past beliefs."
- "... and, I release the need to feel sad, depressed, or any other negative emotion which holds me out of alignment with what I truly want."

This exercise is very helpful. Remember, you may have to revisit this exercise any time a new desire comes into your life and you are wondering why it hasn't manifested yet. You see, the universe always answers you, every time. If you are not receiving, it is only because you are not allowing it.

A healthy life is a balanced life. This is a familiar and comforting image to all of us. Have you ever had a severe inner ear infection? If you have, then you know what it feels like to have your whole world off balance. The world seems to whirl around and you feel completely disoriented. The experience of disorientation can be thrilling, but for the most part, you do not want to be out of balance. Each one of us seeks balance in our lives.

A well-balanced life includes both physical and mental aspects. Living a well-balanced life means balancing your journey to fitness. You have to make adjustments and choices in your lifestyle, if you want to live a fulfilling and healthy life.

> *"Live every day as though it is your last!"*
>
> —**Zig Ziglar**

It would be very easy to live a balanced life in a world with no temptations such as alcohol, junk food, or smoking. What if you could sit down and write the story of your life, making it as healthy as you want it to be? What would you be like? What would be necessary for you to live this life? Much of what happens in your life you have control over; you are not just a helpless person, manipulated by your negative inner talk or those around you. You are able to make choices and decisions to shape your health.

Create a Vision of What You Want Your Life to be Like

Create lasting change in your life by writing down a vision of what *your* ideal life would be. We also have a vision board in our kitchen that we look at every day where we cut out pictures of our dream house, dream car, places we want to visit, fit-looking bodies and sports we want to try. It is motivating to look at each day, and we get excited!

To change your life from where you are today to something better, you must first be able to see what sort of life you want.

Once you can see the sort of life you desire, your mind will lead you in the right direction to achieve it. The most important thing is to trust this process. Unless you believe in it, it won't work for you. Try it for just 14 days. You'll see it really works.

Here's What to do Now

Step 1. Grab a blank piece of paper, or your journal, and write a a vision of your ideal life as you would like to see it in 12 months using the list below.

1. Your purpose in life
2. The people you meet and have around you
3. Your ideal weight and how you feel
4. The exercises you do each day and the food you eat

Step 2. Re-write this vision of what you want your life to be like every night for 14 days or more. The longer you do it, the more you'll imprint this picture in your mind and the more you'll start to believe it is possible for you. Now you are getting closer to making this visualisation a reality.

Step 3. Do it. Take action now. Act on your dreams. Do the things you know are right for you. Only confident, positive action can ultimately change your life for the better.

Important tip:

One very important tip is that you must write in the present! For example, say, *I am*, not I will be; *I live in*, not I will live in; *I feel*, not I will feel; and so on.

Remember, that your thoughts shape your actions, and your actions shape your destiny and your life. If you want to change your life, you must first change your thoughts. The way you change your thoughts is by creating a written vision of what you want, and reading it often. Your mind and thoughts will soon align with your vision and start creating your new reality. For you to achieve any success in your life, you must think it first and then do it second. The *do it* is all about action.

Every morning in Africa, a gazelle wakes up. It knows it must run faster than

the fastest lion or it will be killed ....

Every morning a lion wakes up, it knows it must outrun the slowest gazelle

or it will starve to death.

It doesn't matter whether you are a lion or a gazelle ...

when the sun comes up, you had better be running!

Chapter 21

– Our 15 Health and Fitness Tips to Live by for the Body You Want

We follow 15 simple rules. These rules help us to maintain championship bodies and live long and healthy lives. These rules are also a summary of this book. If you follow these rules you will have amazing results.

1. Drink two litres of filtered water every day.

- Dehydration will make you crave sugar, feel tired, hold fluid, and will stop you from losing weight. A good water filter is essential.

2. Exercise everyday for at least 40 minutes.

- This works out to be approximately five hours out of your whole week – not much when you think about it.
- Book it into your diary, just like you would a meeting.

- Exercise is great for stress relief, losing weight, self-esteem, and it will become a habit.
- Get outside, walk. You don't have to go to a gym to exercise, get fresh air and sunlight!
- Follow our *84 Day Body Challenge Action Manual f*or motivation.

3. Avoid sugar, white flour, carbonated drinks and trans fats.

- Sugar and white flour are loaded with empty calories and will not even fill you up – cakes, pastries, white bread, and chocolate. Once in a while is okay, but not every day!
- Soft drinks have 13 teaspoons of sugar, diet drinks aren't any better as they are loaded with aspartame which is a toxin and lowers serotonin feel good hormones.

4. Get a good night's sleep – at least eight hours every night.

- Don't eat a heavy meal before you sleep.
- Try camomile tea after dinner to relax the body and mind. Half a teaspoon of honey is a great sweetener. No caffeine or tea before bed – you are trying to put the mind to sleep, not wake it up!
- Exercise after work to alleviate stress and calm the mind.
- Try a Nikken™ magnetic mattress – it increases your REM deep sleep and can help alleviate sore joints, tight muscles or headaches.

5. Consume 92 essential nutrients every day.

- Get nutrients in food or as a whole-food supplement.
- Take spirulina and barley grass everyday
- Go back and read chapter 13 on supplements again.
- Refer to www.fitnesskick.com.au for quality supplements we recommend.

6. Use natural products as often as possible to promote health.

- Quick-fix pills like painkillers for a headache are toxic to the body.
- There is a reason for the headache in the first place!
- Start using natural therapies such as massages, herbal remedies, herbal teas, magnetic products, alkaline green supplements, and filtered water that are going to fix the problem naturally rather than putting toxins into your body.

7. Maintain proper pH balance in the body.

- Stress, alcohol, smoking, processed foods, dehydration, lack of sleep, too much protein, and too much exercise are all acid-forming.
- Read chapter 11 - Eat Green Stay Lean again and start living an alkaline lifestyle today.

8. Cleansing the internal organs.

- We clean the outer body every, day but we hardly ever touch the internal body – which is more important!
- Drinking three to four litres of filtered water with fresh fruit and veggie juices over a few days will also help cleanse you out. A mixture of fresh carrot, celery, apple, beetroot, and ginger served with ice is our favourite.
- Have a break from dairy and wheat for a week – your digestion system will love it!
- Do a soup diet for a few days to cleanse the digestive system. Mix vegetables, lentils, chicken stock, celery, leeks, chilli, spinach into a saucepan and cook. Blend until smooth. Great to keep in the refrigerator for snacks and dinners.

9. Eat smaller meals more often.

- Capacity of a normal human stomach is 350 to 450 ml. Most people eat 5-10 times this and stretch their stomachs. Eating small meals also improves digestion and this is necessary for losing weight.

10. Never eat carbohydrates alone.

- Carbohydrates digest really quickly and also create a huge insulin hit, which causes you to be hungry within an hour.
- Always combine carbohydrate meals with an essential fat or protein.

- Dinner time must be your lightest meal of the day. Never eat carbohydrates at night; always have a protein source with vegetables or salad.

11. Take 30 seconds to boost your energy every morning.

- There is a hormone in your body called Melatonin. It is sometimes called your sleep hormone. The longer your eyes are exposed to darkness, the greater the release of this hormone in to your body, creating a deeper sleep.
- When you wake up, you MUST expose your eyes to natural sunlight OR bright light (heat lamps in the bathroom work well) within five minutes of waking up for at least 30 seconds. This drastically reduces the melatonin in your body, you will notice the drowsy and tired feeling you usually get in the morning fading away as your body feels more and more energized.
- First thing in the morning, go for a brisk walk, making sure you do not wear sunglasses so you can expose your eyes to natural sunlight while you walk. If you do not have time for a walk, we always make sure we go outside for a stretch in the sunlight. It only needs to be for one to two minutes. We also have a dawn simulator lamp for our alarm clock, so we wake up to a bright light that gradually gets brighter rather than waking up to the alarm or music.

12. Take ginger for better circulation and better looking legs!

- Ginger has been used for health problems since ancient times. It has antioxidant, immune-building, and anti-inflammatory properties. Always choose fresh ginger over dried ginger whenever possible because it has far stronger healing powers. We use ginger for a variety of reasons – joint pain, increased circulation, decreased fluid, and cellulite in the legs and hip region. According to Chinese medicine, ginger is a warming food, so it is great for turning on the digestive fire for better digestion and elimination.

- Ginger is also amazing for helping to move fatty deposits from legs and hips by increasing circulation in those areas. According to our Chinese medicine therapist, if the tops of your legs and backside are cold to touch, it means the circulation is stagnant and blocked in those areas.

- Follow this ginger tea recipe to increase circulation and help tone up your legs and bottom: Cut up finely a palm-size ginger root and crush with a knife. Bring two litres of water to a boil in a large saucepan and add the ginger. Simmer for one hour then let it sit for one hour. Drink one to two cups of hot ginger tea every day. Keep in a glass bottle in the fridge and reheat when needed.

- According to traditional Chinese medicine, other warming foods that can help with increasing circulation in the body are: oats, parsnips, anchovies, cooked vegetables, stews, cabbage, coconut, avocado, lentils, kidney beans, sweet potato, nuts, seeds, fish, chicken, garlic, cumin, cinnamon, and sea salt.

- Daily slapping also gives your circulation a boost and speeds up the action of your lymphatic system, which gets rid of stagnant waste products in your lower body. Slap your legs and bottom with your hands until your legs are red and slightly itchy.

13. Always take protein AFTER a workout.

- Important for muscle recovery and developing a lean muscular body.
- If you don't feel like eating a meal, then have a whey protein shake.
- Protein is so important to achieving a lean body that we dedicated a whole chapter to it, chapter 15.

14. Positive mental attitude.

- Read books and listen to tapes and CDs while driving. Great speakers and authors we listen to are Wayne Dyer, John DeMartini, Jim Rohn, Tony Robbins, and Bob Proctor.
- Set goals for yourself and put them where you can see them! Cut out pictures of what you want in your life and put them up on the wall. We have pictures of houses we love, places we want to visit, fit bodies, and motivating affirmations.
- Hang around people that build you up and make you feel good – not bring you down.

15. Eat an alkaline food at every meal

- This is the most important tip out of all of them and one we stick to 100%.
- First of all go back and read the acid alkaline list in the Eat Green Stay Lean chapter 11 and make sure you include an alkaline food with every meal.
- If you are finding this hard, and even we do, then it is essential that you take a good quality barley grass or spirulina supplement.
- See www.fitnesskick.com.au for our recommendations.
- Remember, when your body is acidic, you won't lose weight!

Chapter 22

– The 84 Day Body Challenge

"Pain is temporary. It may last a minute, or an hour, or a day, or a year but eventually it will subside and something else will take its place. If I quit, however, it lasts forever. That surrender, even the smallest act of giving up, stays with me. So when I feel like quitting, I ask myself which would I rather live with?"

—Lance Armstrong

Introducing our *Action Manual*

The most crucial of all areas to master in your life is to become dedicated to a goal and stick 100% to the plan, until it is finished. Many people get motivated to make a change in their diet and exercise regime, become educated in regards to their new health plan, start for a few days, even a few weeks and then stop. We have found that people's intentions are always good, but the systems they were on failed.

We are here to help you keep on track with our proven *84 Day Body Challenge*. It is a separate *Action Manual* to this book, and if you follow the step-by-step process, then you will succeed.

Now you should be motivated to accomplish your goals and educated on how to achieve them. There is only one thing left to do – take ACTION.

As Monica and I were writing this book and working on the *Action Manual*, many people asked how we found the time to get it done. How do we have the time to run four businesses, develop an online website on nutrition, study for two home courses for six hours a week, work out every day for an hour, personally train 30 clients, take eight exercise classes every week, travel and teach in schools all over the state, run health seminars, give speeches, keep our marriage strong, sleep, and still have time to write a book?

Our answer is action. We have goals and dreams we would like to achieve in our lives and as long as we are working on them, even if it is a little bit each day, the day will come when that goal is completed.

Imagine if you just improved a little bit each day – even 1%. You made a commitment to yourself to improve on what you did yesterday by just 1%. It doesn't appear to be much, but it is a formula that can be life changing. By applying this to your training, diet or career, it can dramatically change your life. Think about your improvement after one or two years.

> *"Champions do not become champions when they win the event, but in the hours, weeks, months, and years they spend preparing for it. The victorious performance itself is merely the demonstration of their championship character."*
>
> **—T. Alan Armstrong**

You cannot succeed in any sport if you do not compete. The same can be said about losing weight, or increasing vitality. You will not see any change if you don't do it. Action is the key to any success; keep doing it until it is done. And when it is done, it is done! You must have daily action by exercising, eating nutritious foods, and having the right supplements.

Change Your Body with the World's Fittest Couple

The subtitle of our book is *The World's Fittest Couple*. Now egos aside for a minute, do we believe that we are the fittest couple in the world? The answer is no. We are sure there is an ultra-fit couple out there that climb mountains, swim up rivers, bench press trees, and shot put boulders. We just happen to be the fittest couple on the world stage, in our chosen sport, which just happens to be called fitness.

We believe this to be true in almost any sport. Are the champions the best at it? No, they are just the best at doing it. This says a lot about action.

The first part of our *84 Day Body Challenge Action Manual* is an easy to read step by step plan of things to do straight away to get your challenge started. We allow six days for you to get prepared before the challenge starts.

The most important part of the *84 Day Body Challenge* are the checklists. By using the weekly checklists, you become accountable in all the areas of your life you need to improve. We have found these invaluable in our preparation for every fitness competition we have entered.

Our house, in the lead up to a competition can resemble a mad scientist's laboratory! We have affirmations, quotes, checklists, goals, rules, motivational posters on walls, doors, mirrors, the refrigerator and even the ceiling of our bedroom. We do this so that we are surrounded and immersed by our ultimate goal and guess what? It works every time. Don't worry if your house starts looking like a grand final locker room – it will only ensure your success and keep you on track.

When you commit to our *84 Day Body Challenge, you will change your body*. This will ultimately allow you to have a better life.

At this point, how are you feeling? A bit excited, a little overwhelmed? Are a few feelings of doubt creeping in? Start visualizing that in 84 days people will be commenting on how good you look, that you look younger, vibrant and full of energy. They will ask you how did you get into shape so fast and you can tell them you did it in only 84 days.

It is called the *84 Day Body Challenge* for a reason. Firstly, it is 84 days of having that goal, that constant thought, that burning desire, that inner drive, and belief in yourself to achieve success. It can be done in 84 days and that's all it takes – and it is a challenge.

We have done this challenge four times as strict as we could at the time. I can tell you now, all four times the challenge was different for both of us. Why? Because things happen out of your control. You will have good days, bad days, lazy days, and awesome days – however you want to label it. All of that is called LIFE.

The first time I did the body challenge it took me 416 days. But I did it. I changed my body because of one reason to compete and win a world fitness title. I did not allow myself to quit. It is that simple: I refused to use the words hard or impossible and just did the very best that I could.

We implore you to do the very best that you can with what you have. Every one of us is unique, with different strengths and different weaknesses. You don't have to be a certain person to complete this challenge, you just have to DO IT.

If you miss one or two ticks on the daily checklists, or you have done every single minute of exercise needed and you miss a day, it doesn't mean you fail and won't get results. The *84 Day Body Challenge* is a system and the closer you can stick to the system the less adjusting you will have to do along the way. The single most important thing is that you don't stop or quit.

We have never completed the challenge perfectly and placed a tick in every box. Never! Not once! But we always got results, every single time, and changed our bodies. We have never quit though and that is the key to success.

Remember, this challenge is the ultimate guide of everything you need to do. If you miss a couple of ticks here and there, BIG DEAL. Miss a lot of ticks and it may take you a little longer, or you can do what we do. Adapt and adjust your training and nutrition along the way. My goal is always to complete the challenge, no matter what. My aim is to get as many ticks as I can, when I do miss one, I will try and make up for that by trying a little harder in that area the next day. The ticks point out where you need the most help. The ticks let you know your strengths and weaknesses, so you can create a plan to address these areas.

My weakness is fitting in all the exercise components and getting enough sleep, while running four businesses. Therefore, I adapt by getting as many ticks in all the other areas, like the food requirements that I find easier. I make up for missed exercise ticks by either doing extra exercise sessions on some days, or giving myself a hard intense session with a training partner or personal trainer. With the sleep, I take naps during the day to make up the eight hours or sleep longer on weekends!

A final note before you read the exercise and eating plan for the 84 Day Body Challenge:

As long as you know where you want to go, and what you have to do to get there, you will succeed. A plane is off course for more than 90% of its journey, constantly adapting to wind currents and turbulence, and it still reaches its destination 99.9% of the time!

Know where you want to go because the *Action Manual* will show you how to get there as it has for thousands of people before you.

If you complete every single tick, and every minute of exercise, then as far as we know, you will be the first. Remember, it is a guide, not a formula; learn from your mistakes and start again, but NEVER GIVE UP!

Chapter 23

Eat Yourself to Health – Eating Plan

84 Day Body Challenge

The 84 Day Body Challenge Eating Plan is divided into two parts:

1. The first 14 days are called the 14 Day Food Challenge.
2. The last 70 days are the Eat Green Stay Lean™ diet.

Weeks One and Two

What is the 14 Day Food Challenge?

We have put together an amazing food challenge that you can do by yourself or with friends, family and workmates. We believe that a clean diet is 80% of weight loss. You can choose to do the first 14 days of the eating plan online, with friends, or do the hard copy weekly checklists in the *Action Manual*. The website to register for the 14 Day Food Challenge is www.thefoodchallenge.com.au.

Eat Yourself to Health – Eating Plan

The aim of the food challenge is to introduce you to alternative healthy foods to replace the unhealthy vices you might have such as sugar, alcohol, coffee, white bread, and junk food.

These foods, in our opinion, make you fat, tired, irritable, sick, and crave sugar. Giving our bodies a rest from the poison found in processed foods and fuelling them with power from living foods allows the body to detoxify and be energised from within ... a perfect foundation for you to complete the *84 Day Body Challenge*

You are not allowed the following things while on the 14 Day Food Challenge:

1. NO alcohol, soft drinks, or cordials
   Alternatives: water, water, water (filtered PiMag™ water is awesome), herbal teas

2. NO chocolate, sugar, or margarine
   Alternatives: avocado, hummus, organic honey (one teaspoon), stevia sweetener

3. NO cakes, biscuits, or pastries
   Alternatives: thin rice cakes, fruit, yoghurt, protein shakes

4. NO junk or fast food
   Alternatives: sushi rolls, chicken salad pita (no dressing), grilled fish and Greek salad

5. NO white bread, pasta, or wheat
   Alternative: rice, rye bread, wheat-free bread, spelt pasta

6. NO coffee
   Alternatives: black tea, herbal teas, dandelion tea, green tea, ginger tea

You must do the following things while on the 14 Day Food Challenge:

1. Drink a glass of water 30 minutes before meals. No drinking with meals as it interferes with digestion of your food, making you feel bloated, and promotes gas!
2. Exercise for 40 minutes every day.
3. Drink at least two litres of water every day.
4. Eat an alkaline food at every meal.

You will be surprised that after a few days of not having a particular food you may not ever crave that food again! The challenge comes with a checklist, and your goal is to complete the checklist of foods to eat and not eat every day. If you cheat, you are out of the challenge and must start again! The first 14 days must be adhered to so your body can cleanse and detox itself.

If you cheat on day five because you eat some sugar-coated junk food then the 14 day food challenge must be started again. If you are on the online program, then you will automatically be sent some important information on what sugar does to the body, and some tips on how to overcome sugar cravings. Then you start day one again, and attempt to complete the challenge once again.

AFTER the first 14 days have finished and you miss one tick, it does not matter. But during the first 14 days if you miss one you must start the 14 days again. This is very important. You must see the first 14 days as breaking old destructive habits and your first little test of discipline. 14 days to shock your body and mind and give you that important break in behaviour and habit. This allows you to make long lasting changes.

Please use the breakfast, lunch, and dinner options listed in the Eat Green Stay Lean™ diet on the next few pages as a guide of what to eat while doing the challenge.

Please note that you can NOT start week three of the 84 Day Body Challenge until you successfully finish this 14 Day Food Challenge.

Weeks 3 through 12

What is the Eat Green Stay Lean™ Diet?

This eating plan is easy to follow and allows you one day off per week. It is not as strict as the 14 day food challenge and can be a diet that you can follow easily for life. It is very flexible and can be used over and over again, using the checklists in the *Action Manual* – just use different coloured pens. Your whole family can even participate just by putting the checklists on your refrigerator.

When we usually discuss a healthy nutritional plan with clients, the most common response is, "I don't think I eat that badly." Everyone's definition of "bad" is different. Our definition is simple. If you have not followed all seven of the food rules every day, then, yes, your eating plan is bad.

The seven food rules you will be following from weeks 3 to 12 are:

1. Drink two litres of water every day
2. Eat five to six small meals a day (meal size is your hand size with fingers spread apart).
3. Never eat carbohydrates by themselves as this creates a huge insulin hit, digests really quickly, and causes you to be

hungrier. Always combine carbohydrates with a protein or essential fat.

4. Include a protein OR an essential fat in all your meals.
5. Eat an alkaline food source at every meal.
6. Do not eat carbohydrates for the last meal of the day.
7. Six out of seven days, every week, eat clean – NO alcohol, sugar, junk food, or processed foods

We have outlined the above rules in a chart below.

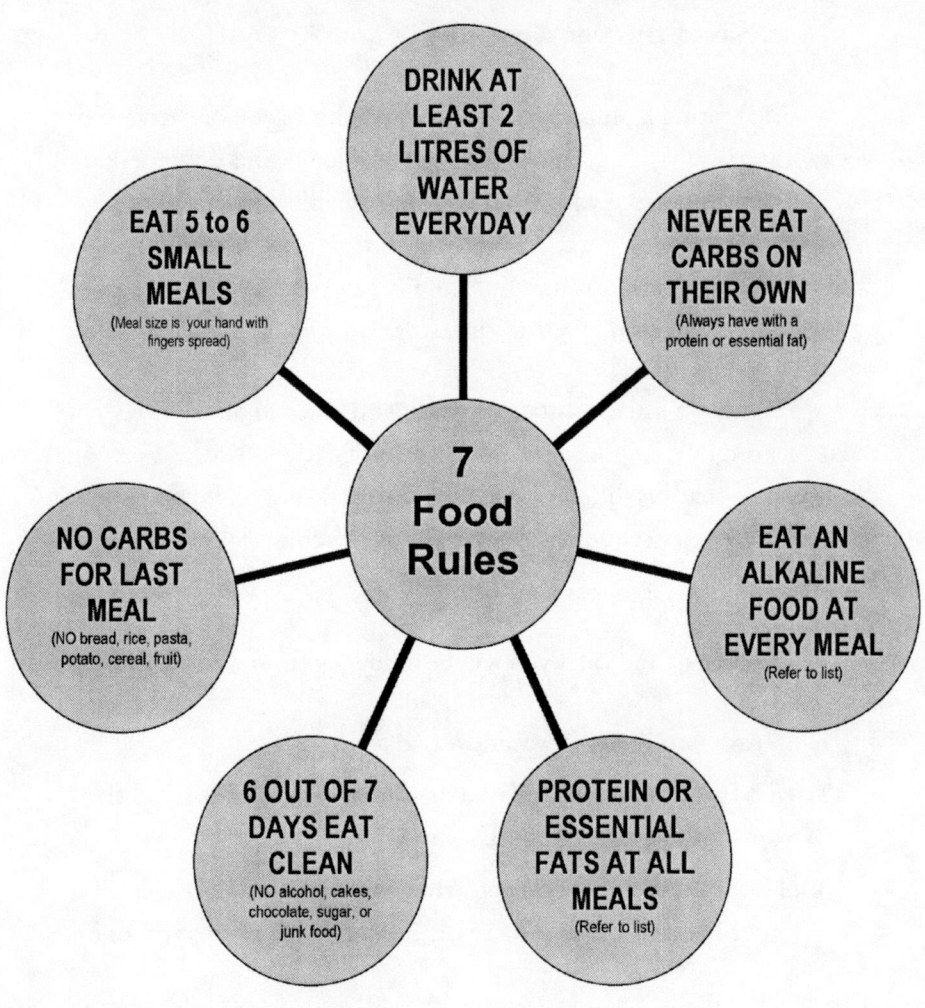

7 Food Rules

- **DRINK AT LEAST 2 LITRES OF WATER EVERYDAY**
- **NEVER EAT CARBS ON THEIR OWN** (Always have with a protein or essential fat)
- **EAT AN ALKALINE FOOD AT EVERY MEAL** (Refer to list)
- **PROTEIN OR ESSENTIAL FATS AT ALL MEALS** (Refer to list)
- **6 OUT OF 7 DAYS EAT CLEAN** (NO alcohol, cakes, chocolate, sugar, or junk food)
- **NO CARBS FOR LAST MEAL** (NO bread, rice, pasta, potato, cereal, fruit)
- **EAT 5 to 6 SMALL MEALS** (Meal size is your hand with fingers spread)

Eat Yourself to Health – Eating Plan

We follow the Eat Green Stay Lean™ diet every day, and we have provided lots of breakfast, lunch, and dinner options for you over the next few pages using the above food rules. Any of these meals can be halved and used as one of your five to six small meals. We actually have two breakfasts every day. We have one at 5.30 a.m., before we start work with clients, and the other at 9:00 a.m., after our last morning client. We pick two of the breakfast options listed. We then do the same thing later in the day. We have an early lunch at 12:00 p.m., then a later lunch at 4:00 p.m.

Dinner for us is at 9:00 p.m. most nights, and is always our lightest meal of the day. An example of our daily eating plan is at the end of this section. As you will see, we eat a lot of food! But we eat it over six small meals and we never go hungry or gain lots of weight. The number one lesson to learn from eating healthy versus eating junk or processed food is that you can eat much more healthy food because it is lower in calories. One upsized burger meal with the lot is roughly the same amount of calories as our whole day's intake of wholesome food!

Any of the dinner options can be used for lunch options. One of our six meals every day is either a protein shake with nuts or fruit, or a mix of barley grass and super juice. Feel free to add your own choice of meals to the list using the seven food rules.

You will not go hungry over these 84 days, and your knowledge of food and how it affects your body shape will be something you can take with you for the rest of your life. You will actually come out of these 84 days with an eating plan that works for YOU for life.

Breakfast Options

| Breakfast Options | Must have
• protein
• carbohydrate
• essential fat
• alkaline | Cook porridge made with a ½ cup of oats and one tablespoon LSA (linseed, sunflower and almond mix) and one cup water in microwave/stove for two to three minutes. Add cinnamon and vanilla protein powder once cooled down. Use stevia to sweeten, if necessary

Protein shake with whey protein, 10 almonds, and a piece of fruit

Protein breakfast shake – mix whey protein, ½ cup oats, one tablespoon LSA mix, and water; mix in a blender or shake and drink

One cup muesli (no dried fruit), one tablespoon LSA mix, 10 almonds plus one cup rice or soy milk, or one cup organic yoghurt |

Breakfast Options	Must have • protein • carbohydrate • essential fat • alkaline	Two eggs either boiled or poached (not scrambled or fried) on two grainy toast with a quarter of a large avocado and sliced tomatoes Two grainy toast with vegemite and quarter of a large avocado spread, with sliced tomato on top Small can of four bean mix, small can of corn, quarter cup low-fat grated cheese – cook in microwave until cheese melts and serve with one grainy toast, quarter of a large avocado, and fresh tomato Two grainy toast with one tablespoon of 100% Nut Butter (mix of almonds, brazil nuts and cashews) French toast – soak one or two pieces of grainy toast in one egg, grill, and then spread one tablespoon of 100% Nut Butter Wellness drink – one tablespoon of barley grass powder and 30 to 60 ml of super juice mixed into a large glass of water, eat with 15 almonds

Breakfast Options	Must have • protein • carbohydrate • essential fat • alkaline	**If going out for breakfast choose the following:** Eggs – cooked any way except fried or scrambled Bread – whole grain, sourdough, or rye only – not white or turkish. Alkaline foods – pick from avocado, spinach, tomato, lemon squeezed over meal, mushrooms, almonds Muesli – make sure it has nuts and no dried fruit – enjoy with yoghurt, limited milk and fresh fruit Coffee – okay, no more than one at breakfast. Green or herbal tea – great choice Juice – if you like your juice, then stick with mainly veggies such as a carrot, celery, beetroot, ginger and a choice of one fruit such as apple, watermelon, or orange juice rather than an all fruit option; drink before your food comes out, rather than with your food for better digestion

Lunch Options

| Lunch Options | Must have
• protein
• carbohydrate
• essential fat
• alkaline | Beef, tuna, chicken, or egg salad sandwich with avocado on grainy bread or rye or wrap with heaps of salad – minus the margarine/butter, mayonnaise and hard cheeses

Two or three Japanese sushi rolls with choice of tuna, salmon, prawn, vegetables or chicken

Large mixed salad with free range chicken or tuna with three crumbled rice cakes in it; or buy a ready-made salad from the supermarket and then add a can of tuna or cut up free range chicken with half a lemon squeezed over meal

Beef or chicken salad if eating out, minus the dressing and one slice of grainy bread with avocado. Half a lemon squeezed over meal

Chicken Caesar salad – NO dressing and NO croutons, with half a lemon squeezed over meal

Most Japanese dishes – but stay clear of deep fried meals

Grilled chicken or steak served with salad or vegetables, no chips |

Lunch Options	Must have • protein • carbohydrate • essential fat • alkaline	Grilled fish with a salad or veggies – potatoes are okay Bowl of lentil dahl served with a garden salad Mix together a can of four bean mix, small can of tuna in spring water, small can of corn, half cup low-fat cottage cheese, quarter of an avocado, half lemon squeezed and pepper, and chilli – serve on three to four thin rice cakes or eat as is Mix together a can of tuna in spring water, half lemon squeezed, fresh tomato, humus dip, a quarter of an avocado and serve on top of three to four thin rice cakes in layers A protein shake with 10-15 almonds and a piece of fruit Medium sweet potato (cooked in microwave for seven minutes) and serve with small can of tuna or half a free range chicken breast with avocado, cucumber and half a lemon squeezed over meal. Tuna, avocado, cucumber, alfalfa sprouts and half a lemon squeezed and rolled up in two mountain breads.

Eat Yourself to Health – Eating Plan

| Lunch Options | Must have
• protein
• carbohydrate
• essential fat
• alkaline | Chicken and sweet corn soup plus serving of Chinese broccoli,

Homemade chicken or tuna pizza: Spread a large, whole meal pita bread with tomato paste, then layer with cut up mushrooms, baby spinach, free range chicken or tuna, squeeze of lemon, half cup grated low-fat cheese, and bake in oven until brown – half a pizza is one serving

Mountain bread lasagne: Use thin mountain bread as your sheets, aim for three layers; layer with cooked free range chicken, low fat cottage cheese, spinach, mushrooms, red pepper, thin sliced zucchini and chill to taste – cover it with foil and cook in the oven

Homemade Soup: Cut up eight carrots, one medium sweet potato, two leeks, and add two frozen packs of spinach, one kilogram frozen beans, two canned tomatoes, 1 large can kidney beans, two cups chicken stock, one teaspoon chilli flakes, one cup dry red lentils, ten cups water and 3 pinches of organic sea salt. Boil in large saucepan, and then simmer for one hour. Blend and serve. One serving is two cups. Keeps for up to five days in the refrigerator |

Dinner Options

Dinner Options	Must have • protein • veggie/salad • alkaline	These dinner recipes are for one person, so please double the recipe if you are cooking for two people. Extra large mixed salad with baby spinach, cucumber, alfalfa sprouts, cucumber, tomato, red pepper and then ADD chicken, beef, fish, lamb or tuna. Make a homemade dressing of one tablespoon flaxseed oil, one teaspoon grainy mustard, one teaspoon of lemon juice, one teaspoon of balsamic vinegar, one teaspoon of olive oil and pepper (shake, stir well and pour onto salad) Chicken Caesar salad – NO dressing and NO croutons Grilled chicken, fish or steak served with steamed vegetables or large salad – no chips, wedges, or potatoes; dressing on side Mix together a can of four bean mix, small can of tuna in spring water, half cup cottage cheese, half a lemon squeezed, pepper, chili, and small can of corn. Serve in large lettuce leaves

Dinner Options	Must have • protein • veggie/salad • alkaline	Free range chicken or turkey breast without skin, 100 grams. Cook in fry pan, or coat with LSA mix & dry herbs, and one teaspoon of olive oil. Bake in oven with zucchini cut into strips, red pepper, and large mushrooms. Squeeze lemon over meal and add chili if needed Omelette: Made with two egg whites and one whole egg. Mix with mushrooms, tomato, and herbs. Serve on salad or steamed veggies. 100g lean beef steak, fat trimmed, garlic and two cups of mushrooms, cook in fry pan. Enjoy with steamed veggies OR salad 100g fresh fish, with ginger, lemon, garlic, organic sea salt, sliced tomato, spinach (chopped) – wrap in foil and cook in oven. Serve with salad. Frozen spinach pack (leave out in the morning to defrost). Mix with one cup of low-fat cottage cheese, pinch of sea salt, and two eggs. Put into small oven dish and bake! Serve with 100g chicken, beef, or fish

Dinner Options	Must have • protein • veggie/salad • alkaline	Veal rolls: Buy thin sliced veal, add cottage cheese, spinach, chilli and mushrooms at one end. Roll up and secure with a tooth pick and cook on oven tray. Serve with steamed green veggies, or salad Chili Con Carne. Cook 200 grams lean beef or chicken mince in saucepan. Then mix in five cups chopped spinach, one can red kidney beans, two cups chopped mushrooms, one cup tomato paste, three teaspoons curry powder, three cups of water, ½ cup red lentils. Simmer for 45 minutes. Serve in large lettuce leaves

Eat Yourself to Health – Eating Plan

Throw out the Trash

Clean out your environment – that is your refrigerator, kitchen cupboards, pantry, car, and workplace – of all 'forbidden' foods detailed below and replace with our 'favourite' foods. We have a saying in our house and at work: *"If it does not have any nutrients, then don't eat it"*

FORBIDDEN FOODS replace with FAVOURITE FOODS

FRUIT Canned in syrup, dried fruit*, orange juice, breakfast juices	Whole fruits, freshly squeezed juices at café or home, frozen fruits (no added sugar) -no more than two pieces per day
CEREALS, GRAINS, NUTS Sugar-coated breakfast cereals, salted nuts, cereals with dried fruit*	Oats, natural muesli with nuts, homemade muesli, wheat or gluten free muesli or cereals, natural nut butter (100% nuts in ingredients)
BREAD White bread, focaccia, Turkish bread, pizza base	Grainy bread, rye, sourdough, whole meal pita (pizza base), mountain bread, wheat free
POULTRY, MEAT Coated, processed meats, deli meats	Free-range chicken and turkey only, leg ham off the bone, sliced corn beef, meats from local butcher, chicken mince made from chicken breasts
EGGS Battery or barn eggs	Free range only
FISH Crumbed or battered fish packaged products.	All fresh fish, canned tuna, or salmon in spring water, or olive oil (drained)

323

FORBIDDEN FOODS replace with FAVOURITE FOODS

PASTA Canned pasta in sauce, white pasta, lasagna sheets	Spelt, vermicelli, or rice pasta – better for digestion; mountain bread instead of lasagna sheets
DAIRY PRODUCTS Ice cream, soft cheeses such as brie, blue vein or camembert	Cottage cheese, ricotta cheese, low fat hard cheeses, yoghurt, feta cheese, goats cheese, rice milk, soy milk
OILS Vegetable oil (never cook with it!), margarine, canola oil	Butter okay; always cook with cold pressed extra virgin olive oil and buy in a dark bottle so it keeps for longer. Coconut Oil. Flaxseed oil is great for salads, cereal, smoothies, but keep in the refrigerator and do not cook with it
SNACKS Any crisps, tortilla chips, sweets, chocolate	Rice cakes, carrots, hummus dip, almonds, organic yoghurt, protein shakes (whey protein), muesli bars with nuts and no dried fruit , nut spread
CAKES, COOKIES, BISCUITS Any product with hydrogenated veggie oils, high fat and sugar, biscuits, crackers, bagels, pastries, cakes, meat pies, sausage rolls, and muffins	Rice cakes
PROCESSED, SMOKED & PICKLED MEATS/DIPS Pickled herring, sausages, bacon, hot dogs, bologna, sandwich deli meats, salami	Feta cheese, olives, hummus dip, smoked salmon, low fat cottage cheese, low fat cream cheese, leg ham off bone, silverside, tuna, salmon, chicken or turkey breast

FORBIDDEN FOODS replace with FAVOURITE FOODS

UNHEALTHY PROCESSED FOODS High fat/sugar foods like cans of baked beans, spaghetti, frozen fish sticks, frozen dinners, packaged cakes, and and cookies	Four bean mix, ready made salads from supermarket (add tuna, chicken, or steak), frozen edamame (soy beans)
*Dried fruit is very dense in natural sugar (fructose) so needs to be cut out	
Remember that low fat products are often very high in sugar, while low sugar products usually have high levels of artificial sweetener	

Sample of Our Eating Plan

- At least two litres of water every day
- Eating every three hours, we would halve our lunch and have mid afternoon; we eat half our dinner at 5.00pm and eat the rest at 9.00pm on long work days.

On Arising

Wellness Drink – one tablespoon of Barley Grass, plus 30-60ml of super juice mixed into a large glass of filtered Pi Mag™ water.

Breakfast/Early Lunch (20 minutes after the mix above OR, if working, three hours later)

Piece of fruit with 10 almonds

or

Piece of grainy wheat-free toast or two rice cakes with one tablespoon of 100% nut spread

or

Porridge made with a half cup of oats, water, two tablespoons of LSA mix, cinnamon

or

Two slices grainy bread dipped in egg and grilled, then; spread one tablespoon of 100% nut spread

or

Two eggs, one egg white, one half cup of oats, three strawberries, two tablespoons LSA mix, cinnamon. Whisk up like an omelette and microwave – it will come out like a big muffin!

or

Two eggs on two pieces of grainy toast with a quarter of an avocado and a sliced tomato

or

Avocado, fresh tomato, and a slice of low-fat cheese on two pieces of grainy toast

Lunch/Early Dinner (before 5 p.m.)

Ready-made salad from supermarket – mix in small can of tuna or a quarter of chicken, a small can of four bean mix, a quarter avocado, half a lemon squeezed and one tablespoon of flaxseed oil for dressing

or

Grainy bread sandwich with salad, avocado, and choice of tuna, chicken or turkey,

or

One cup of cooked brown rice mixed with small can of tuna, four bean mix, half a lemon squeezed, and a quarter of an avocado

or

Three Japanese Sushi rolls – choose from salmon, chicken, tuna, beef, egg, salad

or

Homemade soup – barley, lentil, celery, spinach, carrot, leek, and tomato

or

Cooked medium sweet potato mixed with a small can of tuna, quarter of an avocado, and lemon

Dinner (mainly protein with veggies or salad)

Chicken breast butterfly – coated in herbs and LSA mix and baked in oven – served with cooked spinach, roasted zucchini, roasted red peppers, and mushrooms

or

Chicken, or steak, or tuna veggie stir fry

or

Omelette made with crunchy sprout combination, and mushrooms with steamed veggies

or

Tuna burgers with steamed veggies or salad

or

Chicken veggie layered lasagne made with mountain bread

or

Chilli Con Carne made with lean steak mince, kidney beans, spinach, tomato paste, mushrooms and served in lettuce cups

or

Homemade soup – barley, lentil, celery, spinach, carrot, leek, and tomato

Snacks

Whey Protein Shake with 10 almonds

or

Yoghurt with a piece of fruit and 10 almonds

or

We eat half of any of our lunch options

or

Wellness Drink

All our favourite recipes are outlined in detail for you in the *84 Day Body Challenge* Action Manual

We still enjoy the occasional glass of wine or beer with meals and live by the rule of eating clean 80% of the time. We make sure we do some form of exercise everyday, so that our body feels balanced. If we do happen to have a few drinks or eat chocolate, it is all about moderation. The other thing we always do, to make sure our bodies stay in balance, is to have our supplements every day, without exception! Then, we know that our bodies are getting all the essential nutrients it needs to function 100%.

Chapter 24

Move It to Lose It – Exercise Plan

84-Day Body Challenge

You only need a minimum of four hours and a maximum of seven hours a week to accomplish the exercise portion of this challenge. This is less than 3% of your week that you need to dedicate towards exercise, so make it a priority in your schedule.

We give a range of exercise times because everyone is at different levels. If you are beginning, four hours a week is plenty to get you started. The maximum goal is seven hours. You do not need to do more than seven hours of *intense* exercise; because you run the risk of overtraining, getting injured, burning out, and affecting your results. It is important that the body is allowed to recover after intense training. A yoga class, swim, ride, or walk can be a good recovery session for some and it could be classed as a training session for others.

It is important to say here that many people mistakenly do physical exercise for aesthetic reasons only: to look good for their wedding day, to look good for summer, to look good so they can meet the opposite sex, and so on. They fail to see the medical wellness benefits of doing physical exercise every day. There are numerous studies, conducted throughout the world, that show a direct relationship between a lack of physical activity and heart disease, stress, cancer, diabetes, anxiety, and depression. When you start seeing exercise as a way to reverse aging, increase energy, and reduce stress, it becomes part of your life. You will finally realise that you cannot live a long and healthy life without it. When Monica gets busy at work and it doesn't seem like she has time to exercise, she has a saying to get motivated "Exercise clears my mind and gives me the energy to power on," over and over. She actually uses exercise to make her day more productive, and to wake her body and mind up in the morning.

If you are worried about where you are going to fit an exercise regime into your life, you need to pay attention to these two points:

- Place a higher value on exercise by focusing on all the benefits it will bring to your health and overall quality of life. Use it as time out from family and work.
- Look at how you are spending your time.

Lack of time is probably the biggest excuse not to exercise. Our prime minister and other world leaders find time to exercise one hour a day with the weight of the world on their shoulders. If they can fit it in, then so can you. What is more important than your health? Without good health, your work and home life, which may seem more important at the time, will slowly start to deteriorate. If you cannot afford four hours each week to exercise, you need to look at your time management and create more time in your day.

If you travel for work, try to book a hotel with a gym and take your gym programs with you. If there is no gym, then use the Fusion workouts or cardiovascular workouts outdoors and in your hotel room. You can have an amazing workout in your hotel room, beach, stair well of a hotel, and any road can be used for a run or power walk. Use the gym stick in your hotel room or park for a great resistance workout. There is no excuse! If you are sitting for the majority of the day in a desk job, traveling extensively for work, or attending many conferences, exercise will give you energy and sharper concentration.

> *"If you train hard, you'll not only be hard, you'll be hard to beat"*
>
> **—Herschel Walker**

Move it to lose it. Break your exercise into 2 x 20 minute intervals if you must, but just do it. There is no quick cure for exercise. The body loves to move, stretch, get blood and oxygen circulating and release endorphins, the feel-good hormones.

The training philosophy we teach our clients is: if you can talk freely, you are not working hard enough; if you cannot talk at all, you are working too hard; and if you can talk, but don't feel like it, you are working at the right level.

It's a WORKOUT, so remember to put the WORK in, otherwise you are just OUT. It is all about the intensity. I see some people in the gym do in one hour, what I do in 20 minutes, – I leave absolutely smashed; while they look like they have been at a café for one hour.

Make sure you stretch at the end of every workout!

Stretching out all the major muscle groups, specifically the muscles you just worked on, is essential for injury prevention, and for relieving tired and exhausted muscles from a build-up of toxins. Stretching can also help alleviate permanent stiffness, chronic pain, and joint discomfort. When stretching, hold each pose and breathe slowly, for at least 30 seconds.

Once you start moving your body every day, you will never want to stop; it will become a habit, something you look forward to doing. In the *Action Manual,* there are stretching exercises with photos that are easy to follow.

84 -Day Body Challenge – Exercise Plan

Our *84 -Day Body Challenge Action Manual* is an easy to follow step-by-step training system that has daily checklists and detailed exercise programs ,with colour photos, showing correct technique. It is all planned to ensure your success. It perfectly complements what you have read in this book and ensures you apply the knowledge in an action plan. The *Action Manual* has a list of cardiovascular, resistance, and our popular Fusion, workout programs, with photos.

Change Your Body with the World's Fittest Couple

Each week you must complete three fusion workouts, two cardiovascular workouts, and two resistance workouts. See below for duration of each session – your choice of time – shorter or longer, depending on your fitness.

Quantity per Week	Workout	Duration
Three	Fusion workouts	40-60 minutes
Two	Cardiovascular workouts	30-60 minutes
Two	Resistance workouts	30-60 minutes

Example of a Workout Week on the 84-Day Body Challenge

Day	Workout
Monday	40 minute Fusion workout
Tuesday	20 minute run in the morning 20 minute dog-walk after dinner
Wednesday	40 minute Fusion workout
Thursday	60 minute lower body weights
Friday	40 minute Fusion workout
Saturday	60 minute personal training session focusing on upper body weights and boxing
Sunday	40 minute Power Walk

This is a brief outline of what is involved for the *84 Day Body Challenge*. It is covered in greater detail in the *Action Manual* which is literally a step by step guide.

So it's time to absorb all the information, reflect on what you have learnt from this book and set a date to start the *Action Manual*.

Final Note

Thank you for taking the time to read *Change Your Body*. If you have found just one idea in these pages that will assist you in living a life of abundant health and wellness then we have reached our goal for writing this book.

The time to take action and live your dream is now. You are ultimately responsible for your life. Your life is like an empty canvas and you are the painter who chooses what picture you end up with. Choose wisely.

May you live the life you have always imagined.

Good Luck!

Matt and Monica

"The first wealth is health."

—Ralph Waldo Emerson

Testimonials

Name: Kerry Lugg
Occupation: Fitness Center Manager, Mother and 2004 Ms Fitness Australia

People often refer to this period in our history as the information age.

Within the Fitness, Health and Weight Loss Industry it could be labeled the misinformation age. There are so many contradictions made and for many people trying to lose body fat, tone up or trying to obtain more lean muscle - getting the correct advice seems an almost impossible task.

People throughout the world are getting fatter and sicker and the media talks about the "obesity epidemic" as a disease that man cannot control. The correct information is just not getting through to the people who really need it.

Now this has all changed ....

Testimonials

A "Health Revolution" has commenced.

"Change Your Body with the World's Fittest Couple", written by a couple with a combined total of 11 world fitness titles – Matt Thom and Monica Wright will provide you with the correct mindset, nutrition information, wholefood supplements and exercises to change your health and wellbeing for life.

Their "84 Day Body Challenge" provides a day to day training diary, food challenge and all of the required preparation, warm up exercises, intensity training tips, warm down exercises and food management to ensure YOU succeed if you make the commitment.

Name: Travis Wiffen
Occupation: Property Developer, Queensland

Matt Thom and Monica Wright have finally released their "Secret to a Great Body" with these two "must have" health and fitness books – "Change Your Body with the World's Fittest Couple" and the "84 Day Body Challenge".

The "Eat Green Stay Lean Diet" on reducing the acidity within your body and making your body alkaline is leading edge and a fascinating – user friendly food management program.

Buy these books and stop a friend, family member or partners, bad eating and lifestyle habits and their terminal path of ill health.

Buy this book for yourself - change your body within 84 days and choose to live a healthier, fitter life in a sexier body!

Name: Mary-Ellen Sweeney
Occupation: Mother, Personal Trainer -partner of an 84 Day Challenge participant

This could be the last book you will ever need to read on how to lose body fat for life! "Change Your Body with the World's Fittest Couple" is revolutionary, inspirational, funny, easy to read and motivational. The "84 Day Body Challenge" program can be completed at your home – outdoors or at a gym and best of all – It actually works!

Name: Tara Knobel
Age: 34
Occupation: Project Manager

I joined Fitness Kick after walking past and seeing a brochure on the 84 -Day Body Challenge program. At the time, I was unhappy with my weight, really unfit, and constantly tired. I thought this was a great way to kick-start my weight loss and fitness efforts, and the fact that it was over a defined period of time really gave me something to work toward.

It's hard to pick one part of the program that stood out from the others – in fact, the holistic and synergistic effects of the diet advice, food checklists, personal training, and my weekly exercise homework, is what really made it work for me. However, what really stood out was how committed the team was to helping me achieve my goals. Whilst I was the one who needed to do the hard work, I felt like I had a whole team of people working for me – my personal trainer, TJ kept me on track with my exercise regime, Monica provided fantastic advice on diet and the whole team at Fitness Kick provided great morale and motivational support as I worked toward my goals.

At the end of the 84-day program, I had achieved some fantastic results (which I now carry around in my bag as constant motivation) and was really inspired to keep going. I am happier, healthier, fitter, and I have more energy. I still have a way to go toward my final goal, but I know I have the support of a great team to help me get there.

Name: Shannon Curley
Age: 32
Occupation: Business Analyst

I had been overweight since my mid-teens, and three-and-a-half years in England and Ireland had certainly done me no favours! In hindsight, a lucky bout of altitude sickness, on my way home from South America shed a few kilograms, so I tried to retain the momentum and attempted various diets over the next couple of years. Alas, these were all to no avail. I just couldn't commit to anything and keep the weight off.

I have NEVER been an athlete. I could barely get up the two flights of stairs at Fitness Kick when I started with my personal trainer, and I thought there was every chance I would die after each session. But, it was worth every bit of pain. The satisfaction from achieving physical goals is a real adrenaline rush, very addictive, and extremely satisfying. A personal trainer coaches you way beyond what you think you can do. If someone had told me two years ago that, I could run over 10 kilometres, do over 70 push-ups in one go, and not just complete the Kokoda Trail, but also enjoy it, I would have told them they were kidding themselves! I could not have done any of it without the belief of my personal trainer behind me. Every session is different, so you don't get bored, and they tailor exercises for you. Exercise is now a part of my daily routine and I miss it, if I get lazy.

Knowing exactly what you are putting into your mouth is crucial to a healthy lifestyle, and two years ago, I thought I knew what I had to do. I attended as many information sessions as I could at Fitness Kick @ Flemington to learn about food. I was starting to think about what I was eating, and the amount of processed food I consumed scared me. Now, I try to write a menu for the week – and my rule at the supermarket is to go around the edge – veggies, meat, dairy (and maybe duck into the aisle for some tuna)! Don't get me wrong, I still enjoy over indulging on fish and chips, wine, chocolate ... the list goes on. But when I go overboard, I know what to do to get back on track. Food challenges are a great motivator. On your own, or as part of a group, they stop those bad habits creeping into, and remaining in, your routine. I have not just learned, but also experienced, how eating healthy food actually makes you feel good!

I still have a way to go in achieving my goals – it is a gradual process. But I am fitter, stronger, and more confident than I have ever been.

Change your body, change your life. I certainly did!

Testimonials

Name: Malcolm Twining
Age: 44
Occupation: Manager

I have worked in the health, fitness, and supplements industry since 1996. I have completed numerous training programs and I have taken the majority of supplements available in the marketplace.

In my opinion, most training and weight loss programs do not work in the long term, a lot of companies do not provide acceptable manufacturing and quality safety checks on their products, and you do not receive the benefits they claim.

In 2007, I caught up with Monica and Matt while I was working as the Corporate Sales and Human Resources Manager at GNC LiveWell Australia. Although, I had worked with Monica Wright before, and I had respect for her and Matt through all their World Title Achievements and Personal Training business Success, I read the draft of their book with a certain degree of caution and pessimism.

However, their book had an enormous impact on me as I was finally reading a book on how to get fit and healthy from a couple who walk the talk in training and exercise, and are not naturally genetically-gifted mesomorphs.

What excited me was that the book can help you establish your personal motivation to become healthy and look great, plus it was also an entertaining read.

My next step was to read and complete their 84-Day Body Challenge, manage my food through their recommended alkaline food list, and take their recommended whole food supplements.

By week 10, I had already lost 10 kilograms of body fat and maintained my muscle density. After week 10, I didn't bother weighing myself anymore, as I was happy to wear some clothes that I could not fit in to for over 10 years and enjoy the compliments from my friends that "you look 10 years younger – how did you do it?"

My result was obtained by completing the fusion workouts recommended by Monica and Matt. I did not attend a gym throughout the 84-Day Body Challenge and used my own body weight, a gym stick, and occasionally, some handheld free weights (I can't wait to see the results when I join a gym this month).

The training programs are easy to understand and complete, whatever your age or body type. However, I had completed other similar training programs, so, without doubt, the point of difference to me was reducing my acidic food intake and making my body alkaline through Monica and Matt's recommended whole food supplements and Nikken water filtration system. After training, a quality protein drink, Fish Oil, Glucosamine, Chondroitin, and L – Glutamine Powder helped my middle aged body (with numerous serious sporting injuries obtained from my younger days) recover to achieve this result. Put simply, the 84 Day Body Challenge works!

Follow the program and all you will lose is body fat and your self-defeating food and drink addictions. What you will gain is a healthier body, a healthier image, and you will become an inspiration to your children, family, friends, and partner.

Testimonials

Name: Barb Adam
Age: 50
Occupation: Principal of a large primary school.

I joined Fitness Kick when they first opened in 2004. I had just had knee surgery and was feeling out of shape and out of sorts. My doctor had suggested my running days were over, and I was feeling extremely depressed. I knew Matt and Monica were opening Fitness Kick through contacts in the fitness industry. The day I hobbled in to have a chat with Matt regarding rehabilitation exercises was the day I started to make positive changes to my fitness and overall well-being.

I am happy to say fitness is now a part of my every day life, and I am back to running 10 kilometres.

Matt and Monica are more than fitness trainers. They have a wealth of knowledge in all aspects of fitness, nutrition, and physiology. At my age, with knee problems, and in my job, I can't afford to get injured.

I have reached a level of fitness I didn't believe possible. My training sessions are also used as stress therapy. My favourite training session is to don the boxing gloves and let it all out! Matt has patiently taught me sequences of movements in boxing which helps to keep me mentally alert as well – a great way to start the week or to off-load the previous week! I don't think I would be able to cope as well physically, or mentally, in my position as principal without the support of Matt and Monica.

Fitness Kick is more than a fitness centre. It is unique in the personalised attention each member is given. The staff greets you by name and are able to expertly build a program that takes you to your next level of fitness without causing pain or stress. The staff ensures each session is fun, but each session is fun, but vigorous, to maximise results, to maximise results. I look forward to seeing my homework for the week between training sessions. My training manual makes me accountable for my progress and helps me to track my results.

Matt and Monica model the values and behaviours needed for a healthy lifestyle by sharing their knowledge, realising the potential of their clients, and developing a positive and respectful relationship with each client.

I love to be able to tell friends that my trainers are four-time world fitness champions!

Thank you, Matt and Monica, for being such positive mentors.

Name: Pat Green
Age: 38
Occupation: Automation Engineer

I was 35, fairly unfit and didn't consider my own health and fitness a high priority. I was probably the typical 35-year-old Australian male. After much badgering by some friends who had been working on their own fitness, I began the Fitness Kick's personal training program.

A little over three years later, I still enjoy training most mornings before work and I am still motivated by the support, enthusiasm, drive, and expectations of the personal trainers. They train me and set my workload every week. They challenged me whether

I'm feeling tired or fit and they help me achieve a level of fitness that I couldn't achieve by myself.

My health and fitness is a priority for me. It's hard not to take it seriously when so many others are supporting me.

Name: Simone Baumgartner
Age: 30
Occupation: National Account Manager
              – Johnson and Johnson

Matt and Monica are two of the most inspirational people I know! I have the privilege of being a member of their gym since it opened, and their unwavering commitment to my goals and attention to my individual needs keeps me coming back. They have created an environment at the gym that makes you want to exercise. Much more than just the programs that are written for each person, Matt and Mon are constantly challenging their members to do more and be more.

With the help of Matt and Monica's personal training, my fitness levels have increased greatly, which has enabled me to do things I never thought possible;, such as complete a 15 kilometre fun run in 2006, and the Teva Challenge (five hours of orienteering) in 2005! Through seminars organised by Monica, such as nutrition talks, and also through speaking to Monica directly, I'm more aware of the effects food and drink have on my body. These are things I would never have learned and goals I would never have achieved without the help of these two dedicated and enthusiastic people!

Change Your Body with the World's Fittest Couple

Name: Clare Cowperthwaite
Age: 33
Occupation: Communications Manager

I made the decision to start looking after myself six months before my 30th birthday. I was at least 10 kilograms overweight then, and I had started to worry about what life would be like if I didn't do something about my health. Would I be 20 kilograms overweight at 40, 30 kilograms at 50? I'd been to plenty of gyms before and, like everyone else, had been on loads of diets, but my problem was always the same. It wasn't losing weight or getting fit, it was staying that way when I felt like I no longer had a goal. I had no idea how much things would change after I met Matt and Monica.

Personal training has unquestionably been the key to staying on track, and the food challenges, and other events, have helped me focus on new, achievable goals. Matt and Monica (and the other trainers at the centre) have proven something to me I never thought possible – that exercise can be a part of life that I actually enjoy, and that by making some pretty small changes to my diet and my mental approach, even I could get, and stay, fit and healthy.

Name: Jeanette Hockney
Age: 34
Occupation: Director

I first enquired about joining a fitness centre around a year before my wedding date and was instantly made to feel welcome after walking through the door of their gym. Not only was the front desk staff informative and friendly, they weren't pushy like other places I'd investigated. The truly personal style of personal training, tailor-made for me and my needs, was just what I needed to kick-start my fitness and health regime. Being a member of a smaller, more intimate personal training centre, you feel like you're part of a team. The instructors all get to know you, people know you by name, and they make you feel like they are genuinely there to help and encourage you.

The diet advice worked, and it didn't take long to see results from the increase in exercise along with an improved diet. The inspirational story of their own fitness successes, and their hands-on approach to their clients are part of what made the difference for me. Motivating me, without me feeling like I am at boot camp, and taking a genuine interest in my journey, encouraged me to succeed.

I achieved my goals of feeling healthier, having more energy, losing kilograms, and overall, feeling better by my wedding day. Trying not to get caught in the rut some can do post-wedding, I am continuing to work on my fitness journey. I have realised the importance of having a healthy diet and regular exercise program as we get older. I also believe that having personal outlets helps us, to balance and cope with the fast-paced, demanding lifestyles we now experience. I no longer see gym time as chore time. It is time out for me to escape from all that the universe throws at me, to work hard, and to walk out feeling great. I thank Matt and Monica for inspiring and encouraging me, and I hope anyone reading this is also inspired to take the steps toward achieving their own personal goals.

Change Your Body with the World's Fittest Couple

Name: Robyn Dawtrey
Age: 35
Occupation: Chef and Manager

Since meeting Monica and Matt and the team at Fitness Kick in 2005, my life has improved and changed dramatically! On a recommendation from a friend, I went to Fitness Kick in search of a personal trainer and gym to help me achieve my goal of competing in a muscle and fitness competition.

From my first meeting with Monica, I knew instantly I had found the right place to help me achieve my goal. I was given relevant written information on what is required to compete as well as dietary and training information to read straight away. I was then introduced to Kerry Lugg who was to be my personal trainer.

I embarked on the 84-Day Food and Training Challenge to reach my goal and competition date. Throughout this time, I kept a food and training diary so that Kerry and I could monitor my progress. This was a really good way of learning to be honest with myself about what I was eating, and when, and also how I felt during the 84 days.

Throughout the entire 84 days, not only did I have Kerry's support and encouragement, but also Monica's and Matt's, too. It made a huge difference going into such a positive environment to train.

Since then, I have competed in two more muscle and fitness competitions because I love the challenge! Through Monica's and Matt's teachings, I have learned much about diet, training, supplements and exercise. For example, I have learned the difference between acidic and alkaline foods, and how they affect my body. I had no prior knowledge of this and it is interesting to learn. I'm so inspired by them, as well as keen to learn more, that I'm going to do my Certificate Three and Four in fitness next year, so I can help others achieve their health and fitness goals!

Name: Mena Pannia
Age: 32
Occupation: Pharmaceutical Representative

Six years ago, I found myself watching a young woman being trained by a personal trainer at my local gym. Pounding the treadmill, saturated in sweat, breathless, and immensely fatigued, she could barely stand; yet she was still smiling as she tried to maintain her composure to take the next step. The trainer's enthusiasm and constant motivation appeared to fuel the woman's energy to keep going. I watched in awe and decided, at that moment, that I needed to be trained by this trainer. His name was Matt Thom.

Six years later and I am still personal training with Matt and he remains one of the most inspirational people I have ever encountered. He instils confidence in his clients to believe in themselves and achieve their goals. His knowledge, constant motivation, dynamic workouts, and encouragement change the way you exercise and perceive yourself. He has enabled me to find strength I didn't know existed and to exercise at a greater intensity, and he has taught me how important nutrition is, and that mental fitness is the ultimate health goal. Matt has become a great friend over the years. It has been a challenging, and sometimes painful, journey. I am fortunate to have shared it with him.

Name: Sally Prince
Occupation: Bank Manager

When I first met Monica, she told me she and Matt were opening a gym. I couldn't see any reason for me to join because I had no one who cared to do it for. Her answer was, "You could do it for yourself." She challenged me to join, which I did a couple of months after it opened.

I started with monthly personal training and now do it weekly. For the last 11 months, I have worked out nearly everyday and have never felt better. My fitness has improved, my body is changing, and I feel stronger, and more confident. The support I receive from the staff is fantastic.

But the most important thing to me is that I used to suffer from very blue periods. Since increasing the training, I feel much happier in myself and my life is much better. Some might call me a gym junkie, but it is a lot better than just sitting around. I am doing something for me to improve my life.

I am thankful for the first conversation with Monica. It inspired me to change my body and changed my life. Thank you, Monica.

Testimonials

Name: Robyn Smith
Age: 43
Occupation: Nurse

I have had chronic backache due to curvature of the spine for almost 30 years. Since meeting Matt and Monica, five years ago, I am pain free, fitter, and more flexible than ever. My personal training manual details my improvement over the years. It is personalized with specific exercises to suit my specific fitness needs. Although, I can never say exercise is fun, Matt and Monica are great with the encouragement and motivation I need to keep going.

For me, exercise and a healthy eating plan have to be sustainable. The food challenges and easy-to-follow menu plans that Monica prepares are designed for eating in the real world. Eat clean for six days a week and on Sunday you can have your cake and eat it too!

Matt and Monica are a great team who have created a gym where the atmosphere is relaxed and friendly. They are genuinely eager for their clients to succeed in their weight loss and fitness goals, and they offer encouragement and support for this to occur.

Change Your Body with the World's Fittest Couple

Name: Bianca O'Donnell
Age: 30
Occupation: Meat Packer

I have played sports all my life, but due to an injury I had to stop exercising for a while. During this time, I put on a lot of weight and lost all my fitness. Thanks to Matt's and Monica's 84-Day Body Challenge and the encouragement and training from their personal trainers, I am now back on track. I've lost a lot of weight and gained more fitness than ever. With Monica's knowledge of nutrition, I now have a healthier way of eating.

Name: Nikki Nadstazik
Age: 30
Occupation: Pharmaceutical Rep.

Every girl wants to look and feel like a princess on her wedding day. I trained with Matt and Monica leading up to my big day in March 2006. Using the 84-Day Body Challenge program, which was tailored to my body shape and fitness level, I used exercise and a great diet to totally reshape my body. The continual positive reinforcement from Matt and Monica made exercising fun and the preparation for the big day easy! I can't thank them enough for helping me look and feel like a million dollars on the best day of my life. Since the wedding, I have kept all the weight off and continue to exercise daily and eat really well. If you have a special day coming up, I can strongly recommend Matt and Monica to help you achieve your goals.

Testimonials

Name: Doug Spoor

Just a quick note to express my thanks to you, and your team, for the support and encouragement over the last 84 days. Within the past month, I have been through international passport control four times in two different countries. The difference between the *new me* and my passport photo from approximately five years ago, is such that I have been subject to additional checks on each occasion. And that is just the shoulders up!

I have gone down two waist sizes in my trousers. I now fit in to Jackets that date back to 1974, when I was in full competitive training – unbelievable. I feel great being fit again!

Fitness Kick is like having the ultimate shed in your garden. All the tools you could possibly want are neatly laid out ready to use. The plans are waiting in the cabinet. Any help you might need is immediately on hand. Just turn up and, if you work honestly, you can build whatever you want.

"This book gives the person wanting to change their body the inspiration and solutions needed to take massive action to have the body and fitness you have always dreamed of. Thank you, Matt and Monica, for sharing your inspirational story, and knowledge, with those of us who wanting to make a change."

—**Clare Tonkin,** *Author of "Good Vibrations"*

"Wow, I will never make or have an excuse not to exercise or eat healthy again. I recommend this book with five stars to everyone who has ever tried to lose weight. This is the only book you will ever need."

—**David Butler,** *Author of "A Hand Up, Not a Hand Out"*

References

We would like to thank the following authors for their knowledge, research, and passion for the health and fitness industry. The knowledge from all the authors below has helped us to live a healthy and fit life. Their books have made this book possible.

Author	Title of Book
Ted Alosio	*Blood Never Lies*, Llumina Press, USA, 2004
Ted Alosio	*Whole Foods*, Brad Huddleston Productions, 2005
Sang Whang	*Reverse Aging*, JSP Publishing, Florida, 2002
Shinji Makino	*The Miracle of Pi Water*, Kosaido Books, Japan, 1994
Anne Marie Colbin	*Food and Healing*, Random House Publishing, USA, 1986
Julia Ross	*The Mood Cure*, Thornsons Publishers, 2003

Paul Zane Pilzer	*The Next Trillion*, Video Plus, USA, 2001
Julia Hansen	*Take Control of your Health*, Rodale Publishers, 1996
Paul Pitchford	*Healing with Whole Foods*, North Atlantic Books, 2002
Ian Heads Geoff Armstrong	*Winning Attitudes*, Hardie Grant, 2000
Manfred Urs Koch	*Laugh with Health*, Renaissance Books, 2004
Theodore A. Baroody	*Alkalise or Die*, Holographic Health Inc, 1991
Herman Aihara	*Acid & Alkaline*, George Ohsawa Macrobiotic Foundation, USA, 1986
Paul Zane Pilzer	*The Wellness Revolution*, John Wiley & Sons, 2007
Kevin Trudeau	*Natural Cures They Don't Want You to Know About*, Alliance Publishing, USA, 2004
Mary Shomon	*Living Well with Hypothyroidism,*, Harper Resource, 2005
Netzer, Corinne	*The Complete Book of Food Counts*, Dell Publishing, 1997
Katch, Katch & McArdle	*Exercise Physiology: Energy, Nutrition, and Human Performance*, Williams and Wilkins, 1996.

References

Edward T. Howley, B. Don Franks	*Fitness Professional's Handbook,* Human Kinetics Publishers, 2007
Allen Elkin	*Stress Management for Dummies,* John Wiley & Son, 1999
Robert O. Young	*The pH Miracle: Balance Your Diet, Reclaim Your Health,* & Shelley Redford Young Warner Books, 2002
Michael F. Roizen and Mehmet Oz	*YOU: The Owner's Manual: An Insider's Guide to the Body that Will Make You Healthier and Younger,* Piatkus Books, UK 2005
Mac Anderson	*The Power of Attitude,* Word Publishing, USA, 2004
Keith Ellis	*The Magic Lamp: Goal Setting for People Who Hate Setting Goals,* Three Rivers Press, 1998
Thomas F. Cash, Ph.D.	*The Body Image Workbook: An 8-Step Program for Learning to Like Your Looks* (New Harbinger, 1997)
Ian Blair-Hamilton	*e-article titled Acid Alkaline Balance on website: www.ionlife.info* Author: ian@ionlife.info

Anthony Robbins	*Awaken the Giant Within*, Free Press, USA, 1992
John Kanary	*Breaking Through Limitations*, Life Success Pacific Rim, AUS, 2003
Napoleon Hill	*Think and Grow Rich*, Fawcett Publications Inc, USA, 1970
Julio Melara	*It only takes everything you've got*, Global Support Network, USA, 1998
Brian Tracey	*Maximum Achievement*, Fireside, USA, 1993
E. James Rohn	*The Treasury of Quotes*, Bookworld, USA, 1993
Willie Jolley	*It only takes a minute to change your life*, GOKO Management, AUS, 1997
John McGrath	*YOU Inc*, Harper Collins, AUS, 2003
Rhonda Byrne	*The Secret*, Beyond Words Publishing, USA, 2006
Paul Zane Pilzer	*The New Wellness Revolution*, John Wiley & Sons Inc, USA, 2007
Jason Winter	*The Jason Winters Story*, Vinton Publishing, USA, 2004
Gary Richmond	*A View from the Zoo*, W Pub Group, 1987

References

Craig B. Larson — *Illustrations for Preaching and Teaching, Leadership Journal, Baker Book House, 1999*

Janet Wiles — *The Memory Book: Everyday Habits for a Healthy Memory, Apple Press, 2007*

John Toomey — http://www.lifebalance.com.au/

Alwyn Cosgrove — www.alwyncosgrove.com

Tremblay, A., Simoneau, J., and Bouchard, C.

Impact of exercise intensity on body fatness and skeletal muscle metabolism. Metabolism, 43:814-818, 1994.

Krebs, Hans, — *Otto Warburg: Cell Physiologist, Biochemist and Eccentric, Clarendon Press, 1981 research,*

Vic Shayne PhD. — *Whole Food Nutrition: The Missing Link in Vitamin Therapy, 2000*

fitness kick

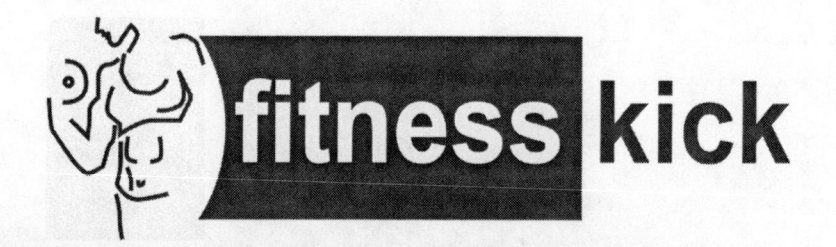

FITNESS TRAINING

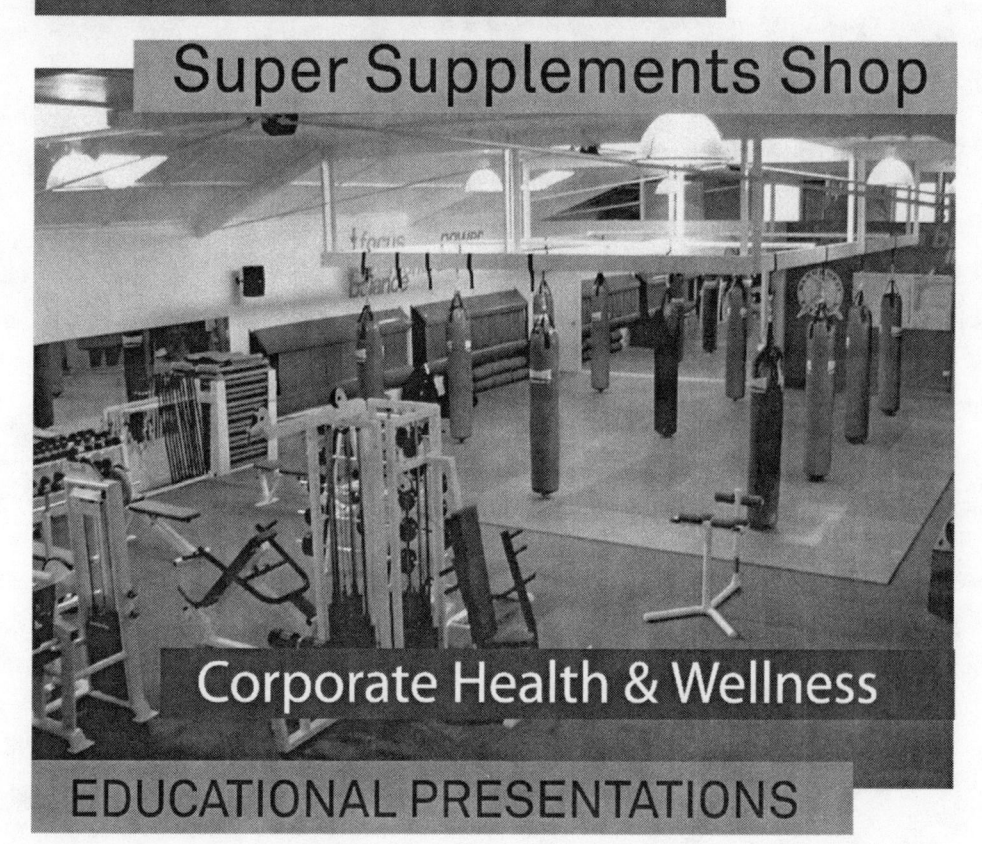

Super Supplements Shop

Corporate Health & Wellness

EDUCATIONAL PRESENTATIONS

www.fitnesskick.com.au
phone: +61 3-9376 8088

TheFoodChallenge

The Online Food Challenge everyone is raving about and getting amazing results… just by eating clean!

Use the Food Challenge to detox, lose weight, achieve the body you have always wanted and get back into a healthy eating routine

Challenge your friends, family, work collegues. Be accountable to each other, it's fun and it really works!

The Food Challenge is totally interactive and teaches YOU what you need to know about food. Are you ready for the Challenge?

START new eating habits, STOP your unhealthy eating habits, Eat Yourself To Health

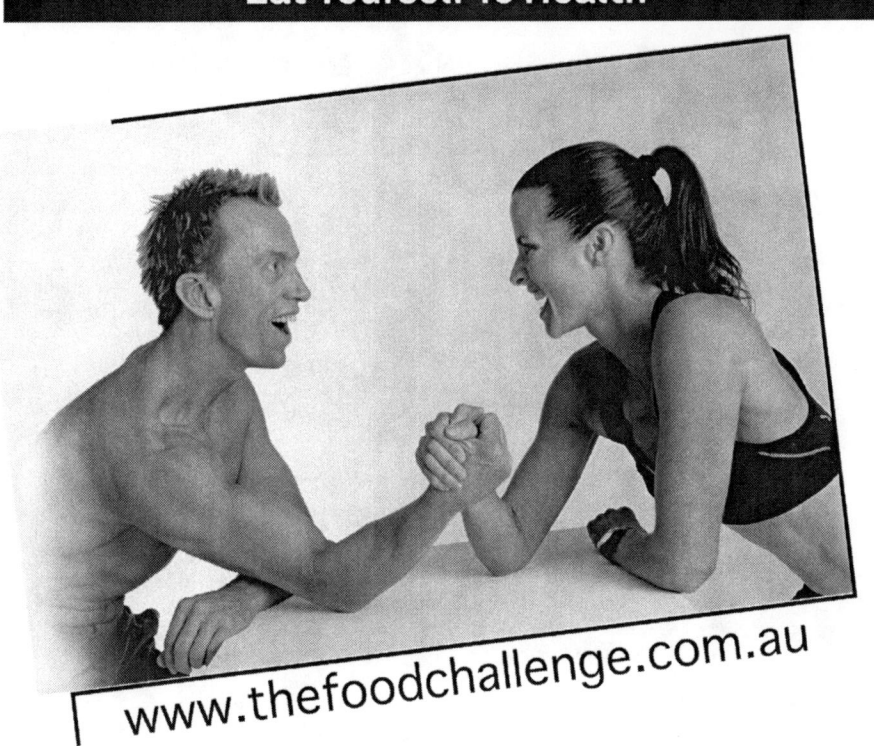

www.thefoodchallenge.com.au

OTHER BOOKS FROM LifeSuccess PUBLISHING

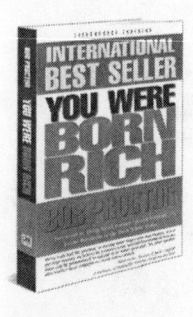

You Were Born Rich

Bob Proctor
ISBN # 978-0-9656264-1-5

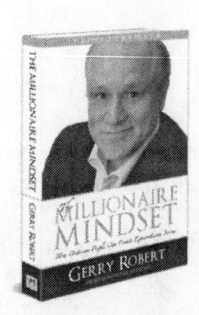

The Millionaire Mindset
How Ordinary People Can Create Extraordinary Income

Gerry Robert
ISBN # 978-1-59930-030-6

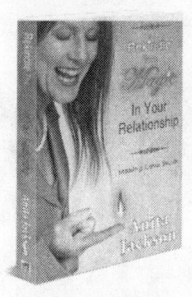

Rekindle The Magic In Your Relationship
Making Love Work

Anita Jackson
ISBN # 978-1-59930-041-2

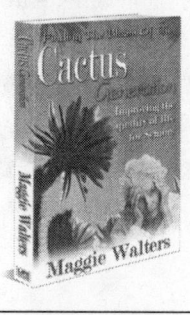

Finding The Bloom of The Cactus Generation
Improving the quality of life for Seniors

Maggie Walters
ISBN # 978-1-59930-011-5

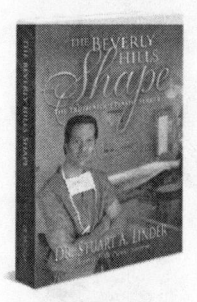

The Beverly Hills Shape
The Truth About Plastic Surgery

Dr. Stuart Linder
ISBN # 978-1-59930-049-8

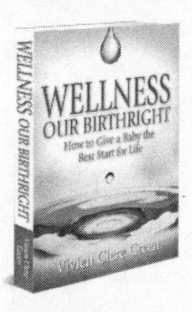

Wellness Our Birthright
How to give a baby the best start in life.

Vivien Clere Green
ISBN # 978-1-59930-020-7

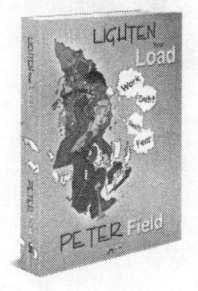

Lighten Your Load

Peter Field
ISBN # 978-1-59930-000-9

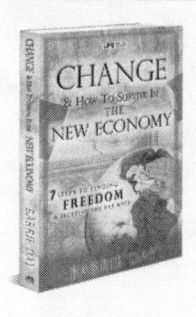

Change & How To Survive In The New Economy
7 steps to finding freedom & escaping the rat race

Barrie Day
ISBN # 978-1-59930-015-3

OTHER BOOKS FROM LIFESUCCESS PUBLISHING

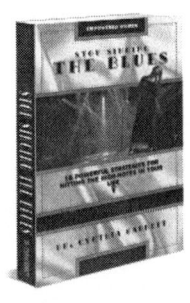

Stop Singing The Blues
10 Powerful Strategies For Hitting The High Notes In Your Life

Dr. Cynthia Barnett
ISBN # 978-1-59930-022-1

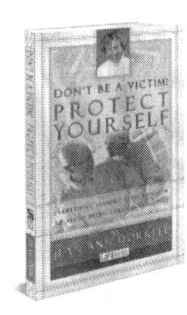

Don't Be A Victim,
Protect Yourself
Everything Seniors Need To Know To Avoid Being Taken Financially

Jean Ann Dorrell
ISBN # 978-1-59930-024-5

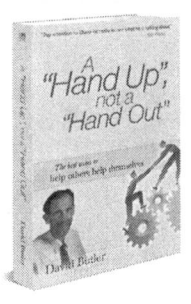

A "Hand Up", not a "Hand Out"
The best ways to help others help themselves

David Butler
ISBN # 978-1-59930-071-9

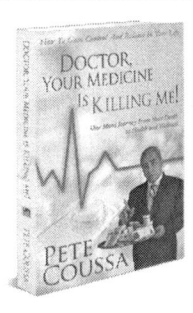

Doctor Your Medicine Is Killing Me!
One Mans Journey From Near Death to Health and Wellness

Pete Coussa
ISBN # 978-1-59930-047-4

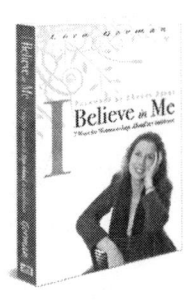

I Believe in Me
7 Ways for Woman to Step Ahead in Confidence

Lisa Gorman
ISBN # 978-1-59930-069-6

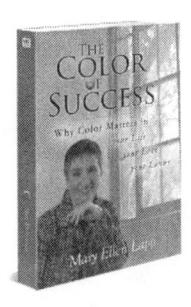

The Color of Success
Why Color Matters in your Life, your Love, your Lexus

Mary Ellen Lapp
ISBN # 978-1-59930-078-8

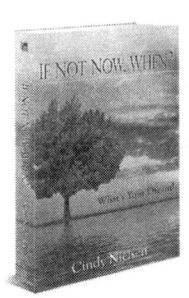

If Not Now, When?
What's Your Dream?

Cindy Nielsen
ISBN # 978-1-59930-073-3

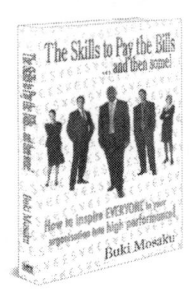

The Skills to Pay the Bills... and then some!
How to inspire everyone in your organisation into high performance!

Buki Mosaku
ISBN # 978-1-59930-058-0

OTHER BOOKS FROM LIFESUCCESS PUBLISHING

The Secret To Cracking
The Property Code
*7 Timeless Principles for
Successful Real Estate
Investment*

Richard S.G. Poole
ISBN # 978-1-59930-063-4

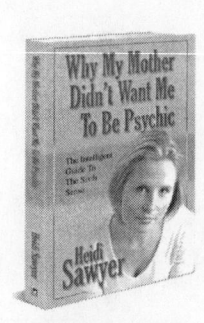

Why My Mother Didn't
Want Me To Be Psychic
*The Intelligent Guide To The
Sixth Sense*

Heidi Sawyer
ISBN # 978-1-59930-052-8

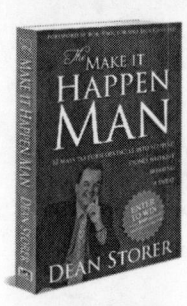

The Make It Happen Man
*10 ways to turn obstacles
into stepping stones without
breaking a sweat*

Dean Storer
ISBN # 978-1-59930-077-1

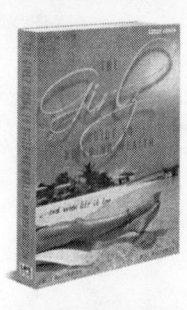

The Girlz Guide to
Building Wealth
...and men like it too

Maya Galletta, Aaron
Cohen, Polly McCormick,
Mike McCormick
ISBN # 978-1-59930-048-1

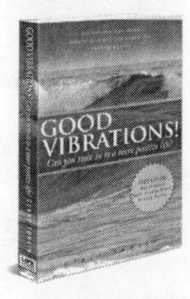

Good Vibrations!
*Can you tune in to a more
positive life?*

Clare Tonkin
ISBN # 978-1-59930-064-1

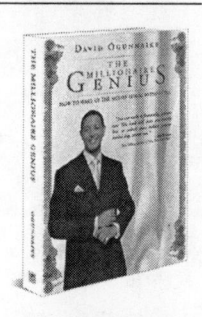

The Millionaire Genius
*How to wake up the money
magic within you.*

David Ogunnaike
ISBN # 978-1-59930-026-9

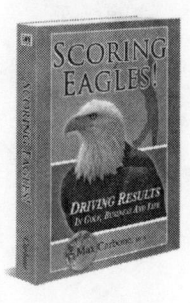

Scoring Eagles
*Improve Your Score In Golf,
Business and Life*

Max Carbone
ISBN # 978-1-59930-045-0

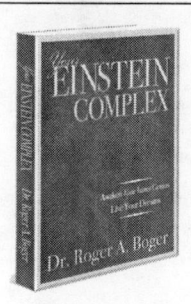

The Einstein Complex
*Awaken your inner genius,
live your dream.*

Dr. Roger A. Boger
ISBN # 978-1-59930-055-9